Sports Medicine
and Musculoskeletal Ultrasound

W0080871

Mouhanad M. El-Othmani
Henry T. Goitz
J. Antonio Bouffard

Sports Medicine and Musculoskeletal Ultrasound

A Pocket Guide

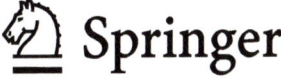
Springer

Mouhanad M. El-Othmani
Department of Orthopaedic
Surgery
Columbia University Medical
Center/New York-Presbyterian
Hospital
New York, NY
USA

Henry T. Goitz
Department of Orthopedic
Surgery
Detroit Medical Center
Detroit, MI
USA

J. Antonio Bouffard
Department of Radiology
Detroit Medical Center
Madison Heights, MI
USA

ISBN 978-3-031-11763-3   ISBN 978-3-031-11764-0   (eBook)
https://doi.org/10.1007/978-3-031-11764-0

© The Editor(s) (if applicable) and The Author(s), under exclusive license to
Springer Nature Switzerland AG 2022
This work is subject to copyright. All rights are solely and exclusively licensed by
the Publisher, whether the whole or part of the material is concerned, specifically
the rights of translation, reprinting, reuse of illustrations, recitation, broadcasting,
reproduction on microfilms or in any other physical way, and transmission or
information storage and retrieval, electronic adaptation, computer software, or by
similar or dissimilar methodology now known or hereafter developed.
The use of general descriptive names, registered names, trademarks, service
marks, etc. in this publication does not imply, even in the absence of a specific
statement, that such names are exempt from the relevant protective laws and
regulations and therefore free for general use.
The publisher, the authors, and the editors are safe to assume that the advice and
information in this book are believed to be true and accurate at the date of
publication. Neither the publisher nor the authors or the editors give a warranty,
expressed or implied, with respect to the material contained herein or for any
errors or omissions that may have been made. The publisher remains neutral with
regard to jurisdictional claims in published maps and institutional affiliations.

This Springer imprint is published by the registered company Springer Nature
Switzerland AG
The registered company address is: Gewerbestrasse 11, 6330 Cham, Switzerland

Preface

Musculoskeletal ultrasound has made a huge impact on the diagnostic and therapeutic care of extremity injury. It allows the clinician a dynamic assessment of pathologic processes, and the patient can even tell the scanner exactly where "it hurts!" So both painful sites and sites of functional loss can be readily assessed, as can ligamentous laxity of joints, localization of cystic formation, tendon ruptures, and the like. It is a tool that can be mastered like any other with practice. Both primary care physicians and orthopedic surgeons alike have championed its value. In the sports world, the portability of these devices has proven their value on the Olympic ski slopes to professional sporting venues. Interested persons can be taught to scan, from athletic trainers to technologists. All have the ability to learn this skill. Ultrasound has proven to be of value not only on the earth in countries around the world, but also "out of this world" on the International Space Station where astronauts are taught the skills of ultrasound, and images of concern are beamed back to clinical specialists on earth.

The motivation for this text is to hold in one place the "tricks and techniques" that have been amassed over a lifetime of dedication to musculoskeletal ultrasound by one individual, namely, Tony Bouffard, MD. He has worked on perfecting his skill and has shared his knowledge in the education of thousands of individuals around the world, from Europe to India; from Asia to South America; from educating Orthopedic Surgeons, Primary Care Physicians, Physician Assistants, Athletic Trainers, and Technologists, to Resident Physicians and Medical Students. He was involved with one of the first medical school curriculums in musculoskeletal ultrasound at Wayne State University in Detroit, to develop the international curriculum and accreditation through the Universidad Catolica de Murcia, Spain. He has been the invited guest lecturer and/or course director to countless national and international meetings and multiple universities from around the world as their featured guest.

I have personally seen the value of ultrasound in my orthopedic practice and in that of my orthopedic peers. Skillful use of the ultrasound transducer can help to make challenging diagnoses very obvious. Moreover, the therapeutic use of ultrasound-guided injections and aspirations can give tremendous relief to those in significant pain, or provide a pathologic diagnosis.

The initial manner in which these pages were compiled was through the diligent compilation of multiple lectures, discussions, and "hands on" courses that Dr. Bouffard was involved with in the training of our Orthopedic Residents at the Detroit Medical Center, Michigan. They were then organized as an easy-to-use guide for understanding and learning musculoskeletal ultrasound.

It is the hope of the authors that you find this guide a powerful way to experience the world of musculoskeletal ultrasound and that you find its "tricks and techniques" useful in your growth with this magnificent clinical tool.

Good luck!

Detroit, MI, USA   Henry T. Goitz

Acknowledgments

The authors would like to acknowledge Daniel Shelton and FujiFilm Sonosite for their support and efforts that facilitated the completion of this work.

Contents

General Overview of Musculoskeletal Ultrasound

General Concepts

1. Musculoskeletal ultrasound applies high-resolution scanning through high-frequency sound waves (3–17 MHz) to produce detailed anatomic images of various musculoskeletal structures.
2. Advantages of ultrasound, when applied to the musculoskeletal system, include the capacity to perform real-time dynamic examination, while allowing the clinician to correlate imaging findings to patient symptoms. The static images obtained ultrasonographically can be complemented with sono-palpation and observing patient's feedback, providing a critical diagnostic tool.
   a. Main additional advantages of ultrasound in comparison to alternative imaging tools include:
   b. Capacity to perform contralateral extremity comparison
   c. Minimal impact imposed by metal artifacts
   d. Portability
   e. Low cost
   f. Lack of radiation risk
3. In addition to the considerably high operator dependency, the main limitation of ultrasound is imposed by the physical characteristics of sound waves as the field of view and penetration are limited to a relatively small area.

© The Author(s), under exclusive license to Springer Nature Switzerland AG 2022

M. M. El-Othmani et al., *Sports Medicine and Musculoskeletal Ultrasound*, https://doi.org/10.1007/978-3-031-11764-0_1

Basic Principles

1. The ultrasound waves used by the machine are generated by applying an alternating electrical current to the transducer, which contains an array of thin crystals that will vibrate and generate a sinusoidal sound wave upon stimulation by the electric current.
   a. This transformation of electrical energy into mechanical energy (in the form of waves) is defined as piezoelectricity.
   b. The range of frequency a single transducer can produce is mostly determined by the material properties and thickness of the incorporated crystals.
   c. The sound waves have characteristic frequency, propagation speed, amplitude, and wavelength, which are mostly determined by the characteristics of the electric current applied.
2. As the sound waves pass through the ultrasonographic gel and into the body, the waves will continue traveling until encountering a change in the density of the travel medium (known as acoustic interface between adjacent tissues with different characteristics), which will lead to the reflection of a portion of the sound wave's energy and allow for the rest to continue deeper penetration.
3. Through a reverse mechanism to sound wave generation, the transducer acts as a receiver to assimilate the reflected sound wave energy and translates the mechanical energy into electrical energy. The ultrasound machine will assess and record the depth of the reflecting structures and the amplitude of the returning waves.
4. The process of generating and recording the sound waves over 7000 times per second allows the machine's software to generate an image of the various structures and traveled medium.
5. The ultrasound image is based on the material characteristic of a specific medium relative to the surrounding medium, and not based on the absolute material properties of the specific tissue. Hence, a structure that is more reflective will appear brighter while a structure reflecting a smaller amount of sound waves energy will appear darker when compared to adjacent tissues.

6. The ability to differentiate two separate structures (spatial resolution) is improved by using high-frequency sound waves, which can be identified by the smaller values for resolution (a 1 mm resolution is a higher resolution compared to a 1 cm resolution).

Scanning Basics

1. Transducer selection:
   a. Determined by depth of target anatomical region.
   b. Frequency and depth are governed by an inverse relationship where higher frequency will have lower penetration depth.
   c. High frequency transducers (10 MHz) have a penetration depth of around 6 cm and can still be used in most diagnostic musculoskeletal examinations.
   d. The curved transducers will typically scan at lower frequencies (2–6 MHz) and used when deeper penetration is needed, while sacrificing the resolution of the produced images.
   e. The small high-frequency transducer (hockey stick) provides similar image resolution and depth penetration as the regular high-frequency transducer; however, it allows for more maneuverability in smaller and curved anatomic regions.
2. Machine settings:
   a. Depth control—controls the desired depth of displayed image and should be adjusted appropriately to include the region of interest.
   b. Focal zone position—focal zone is defined as the point at which the ultrasound beams narrow the most prior to widening as they travel deeper, and should be positioned at the same location as the target structure for optimal lateral resolution.
   c. Frame rates—ability to identify the spatial position of a structure at any point in time, and a higher frame rate is required for rapidly moving structures (mainly in dynamic testing).

    d. Gain control—allows the amplification of all the wave sounds reflected from a structure and should be adjusted to optimize brightness of the target region.

3. Scanning principles:

    a. As ultrasound generates a 2-dimensional image of a 3-dimensional structure, key anatomic areas and all pathology should be generally documented in two orthogonal planes. Those planes are the long axis (LNX) and short axis (SAX) relative to the target structure. These planes can also be referred to as the longitudinal and transverse anatomic planes of the structure being assessed.

    b. Various scanning techniques, including sliding, heeltoeing, tilting, and rotating the transducer are generally applied to optimize the image of the scanned structures and to avoid anisotropy.

        i. Anisotropy is defined by the abnormal dark appearance of a normal structure due to the reflection angle of the sound waves away from the receiver. As sound waves encounter an anatomic structure, waves hitting the structure at a perpendicular angle will be reflected, captured by the receiver, and subsequently processed to provide the image. However, waves that are meeting the structure of interest at an angle will be reflected away from the transducer and will be displayed as a hypoechoic (or dark) area in the image, leading to anisotropy.

        ii. As some pathologic processes have a characteristic hypoechogenicity on ultrasound examination, anisotropy (an operator-dependent artifact) might lead to false positive diagnosis, and should be avoided.

        iii. The manipulation of the transducer through the aforementioned maneuvers might help with directing the sound waves in a perpendicular fashion to the structure of interest and hence avoid anisotropy.

    c. Maintain full control of the transducer probe using the "hands-on" approach, which is achieved through a firm grip on the transducer, and stabilization of the transducer on the patient's body by using the fingers and the hand as a foundation for transducer control and manipulation.

Scanning Approach

1. All joint areas have been divided into specific regions. In general, when performing a diagnostic examination of the shoulder joint, all structures on the protocol are evaluated, constituting a complete evaluation of the shoulder region. This approach is most practically applicable to the shoulder, as a full diagnostic examination needs to be undertaken prior to determining the etiology of presenting symptoms. In the case of other joints, a diagnostic ultrasound may involve examination of the structures within 2 or more regions (e.g., a complete diagnostic ultrasound of the lateral elbow region, complete diagnostic ultrasound of the posterior ankle region), or be targeted to a specific anatomic structure (e.g., a limited diagnostic ultrasound of the common extensor tendon of the lateral elbow region, or limited examination of the plantar fascia).

2. Performance of a complete diagnostic ultrasound examination of a specific body region (e.g., shoulder, lateral elbow, posterior knee, dorsal wrist) generally includes evaluation of all structures on the appropriate checklist (e.g., lateral elbow region checklist). The regional protocol checklists serve as a foundation and navigation for the examination. Practitioners should supplement the regional examination with additional views and diagnostic maneuvers as clinically indicated.

3. Documentation for a diagnostic ultrasound examination should include the indication for the examination, the specific structures examined, and the interpretation of findings (by the interpreting practitioner). Pictures or videos (for dynamic maneuvers) of all examined structures should be saved in a readily retrievable format.

4. Comparison with the contralateral side should be performed as indicated. Standard contralateral comparisons are not considered the standard of care.

5. When scanning, consider:
   a. Static images
   b. Dynamic images
      i. May improve conspicuity of pathology

      ii. Detection of pathology only seen dynamically (e.g., snapping tendons, joint laxity)

     iii. Methods

        1. Active motion (e.g., joint range of motion (ROM), muscle activation)

        2. Passive motion (e.g., passive ROM, pressing on tendon or muscles with your fingers or hand)

        3. Compression

   c. Doppler evaluation

6. With respect to masses and fluid collections, the following should be documented:

   d. Location and relationship to surrounding structures

   e. Size (three dimensions)—list dimension with largest size first, the dimension perpendicular to this as second, and the remaining dimension third

   f. Presence or absence of Doppler flow, as well as location (within the mass or on the periphery of the mass)

   g. As indicated, shape, margins, echo-signature, and compressibility

7. For interventional procedures, the physician should plan the procedure to optimize needle visualization while avoiding sensitive structures and minimizing the distance to the target. Pre-procedure planning should include documentation of the target site, including assessment for Doppler flow in the region of the projected needle path. Optimally, images of the actual procedure as well as post-procedure images should be archived. The diagnostic scan performed as part of procedural planning is considered part of the procedure and is not a separately billable service.

Ultrasound of the Shoulder

2

- Transducer: Linear-array and/or curved linear-array.
- Variable applied pressure with transducer.
- Doppler deployed for all blood vessels and suspected lesions.

Anterior Shoulder Region

- *Long Bicipital Tendon and Biceps Brachii*
  - Patient Position: seated with hand supinated resting on thigh.
  - Examiner Position: seated, shoulder-to-shoulder with patient.
  - Probe Placement: anterior deltoid, and below acromion.
  - Bony Acoustic Landmark(s): coracoid process, greater-and-lesser tuberosities, then bicipital groove.
  - Target: the long bicipital tendon will be found in the bicipital groove between the greater and lesser tuberosities, and appears as a hyperechoic and fibrillar structure (Fig. 2.1a, b).
  - Scan-Sweep: the extra-articular segment of the long bicipital tendon can be traced proximally from outlet portion to distally across the myotendinous junction (MTJ) into the biceps brachii.

© The Author(s), under exclusive license to Springer Nature Switzerland AG 2022

M. M. El-Othmani et al., *Sports Medicine and Musculoskeletal Ultrasound*, https://doi.org/10.1007/978-3-031-11764-0_2

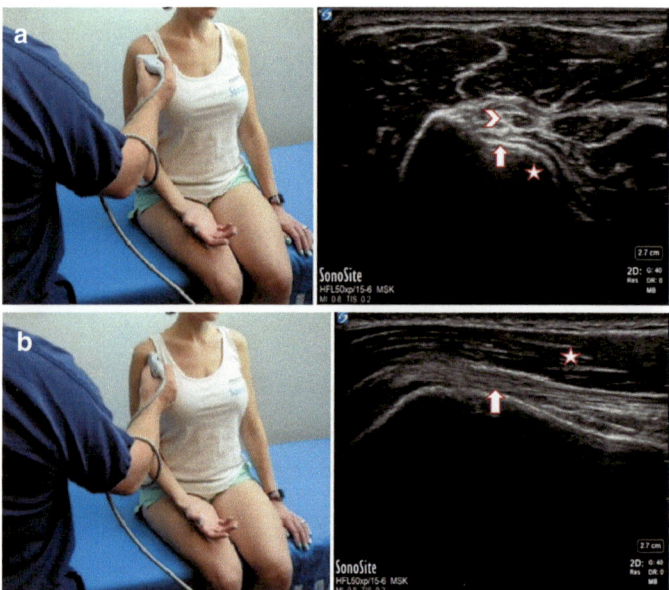

Fig. 2.1 Long Bicipital Tendon. Long head of the biceps brachii tendon (Sax and Lnx). Sax view (**a**) and Lnx view (**b**) of transducer placement and corresponding ultrasound images. (**a**) Long head of the biceps brachii tendon (chevron) in the bicipital groove (arrow). Lesser tuberosity indicated by star. (**b**) Long head of the biceps brachii tendon (arrows) deltoid muscle (star)

- *Pectoralis Major Tendon*
    - Patient Position: seated with hand supinated resting on thigh.
    - Examiner Position: seated, shoulder-to-shoulder with patient.
    - Probe Placement: Proximal-third upper arm, medially.
    - Bony Acoustic Landmark: lateral lip of bicipital groove, proximal humerus.
    - Target: pectoralis major tendon footprint and MTJ. The tendon can be seen as a fibrillar hyperechoic structure on Lnx (Fig. 2.2a, b).
    - Scan-Sweep: pectoralis major footprint to MTJ.

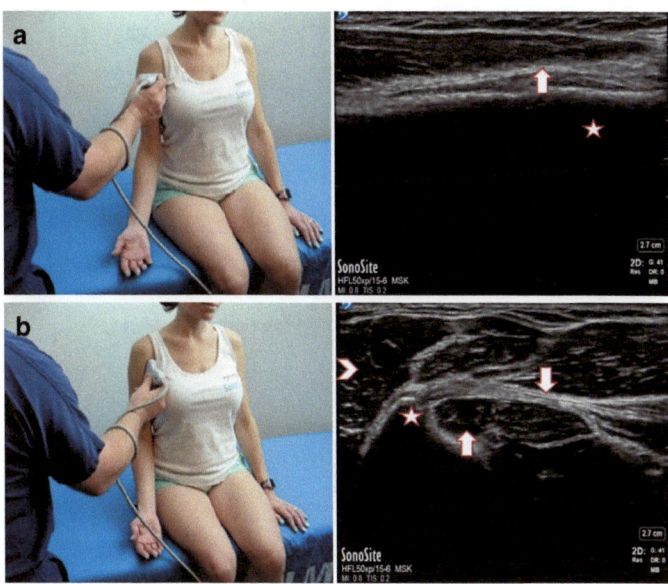

Fig. 2.2 Pectoralis Major Tendon. Pectoralis major tendon (Sax and Lnx). Lnx view (**a**) and Sax view (**b**) of transducer placement and corresponding ultrasound images. (**a**) Pectoralis major tendon (arrow) and the humerus (star) can be seen. (**b**) Pectoralis major tendon (down arrow) attaching at the lateral aspect of the bicipital groove (star). The deltoid (chevron) and biceps (up arrow) are also noted

- *Subscapularis Tendon and Muscle*
  - Patient Position: arm resting alongside body, then in external rotation with the elbow flexed at 90°.
  - Examiner Position: seated, shoulder-to-shoulder with patient.
  - Probe Placement: deltopectoral groove, below distal-third clavicle.
  - Bony Acoustic Landmark(s): bicipital groove, lesser tuberosity, humeral head, coracoid process, and anterior deltoid shelf.
  - Target: subscapularis footprint, tendon midsubstance, MTJ, and subcoracoid recess. On Lnx view, the subscapularis ten-

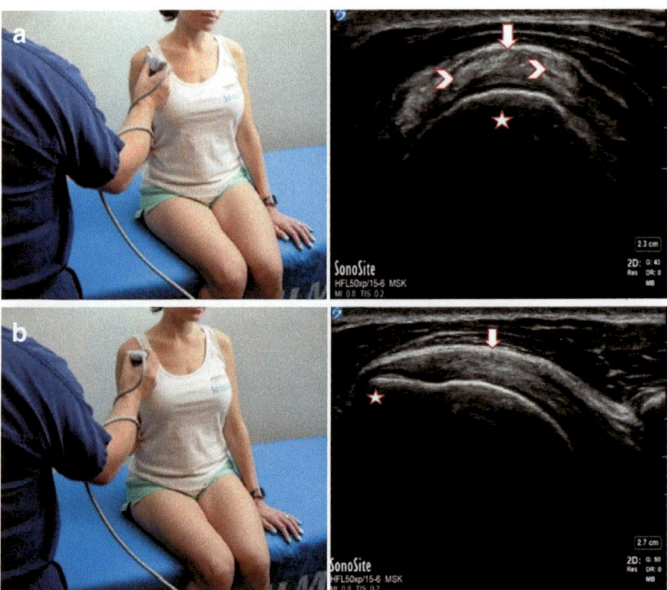

Fig. 2.3 Subscapularis Tendon and Muscle. Subscapularis tendon (Sax and Lnx). Sax view (**a**) and Lnx view (**b**) of transducer placement and corresponding ultrasound images. (**a**) Subscapularis tendon (arrow), humeral head (star) are highlighted. The hypoechoic tendon (chevrons) appearance from anisotropy when sound beam is not perpendicular to the tendon. (**b**) Subscapularis tendon (arrow) and the lesser tuberosity (star) can be seen

don will be anterior coursing towards the lesser tuberosity, and appears as a hyperechoic and fibrillar structure (Fig. 2.3a, b).
- Scan-Sweep: windshield wiper motion from superior margin of tendon to inferior portion, and from footprint to MTJ.
- *Rotator Cuff Interval*
  - Patient Position: seated, now with palm on ipsilateral buttock (the William "Bill" Middleton position).
  - Examiner Position: seated, shoulder-to-shoulder with patient.
  - Probe Placement: lateral to coracoid process.

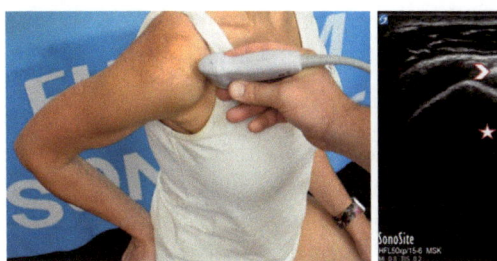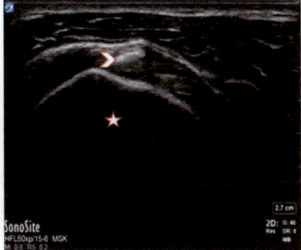

Fig. 2.4 Rotator Cuff Interval. Rotator interval in Sax view of transducer placement and corresponding ultrasound image. Long biceps brachii tendon (arrow) and humerus (star) are highlighted

- Bony Acoustic Landmark(s): bicipital groove at outlet segment, humeral subchondral plate, and apex of lesser tuberosity.
- Target(s):
    Tendons: long bicipital tendon in the hiatus between leading-edge of supraspinatus and superior margin of subscapularis (Fig. 2.4).
    Ligaments: lateral and medial limbs of the coracohumeral ligament, superior glenohumeral ligament, rotator cuff pulley, and capsule. The coracohumeral ligament is located in the roof of the interval and the anterior glenohumeral ligament in its anterior aspect.
- Scan-Sweep: cranio-caudal along outlet segment of long bicipital tendon.
- *Dynamic exam for long bicipital tendon subluxation and subcoracoid impingement (simultaneous)*
    - Patient Position: seated with hand supinated resting on thigh.
    - Examiner Position: seated, shoulder-to-shoulder with patient.
    - Probe Placement: anterior deltoid, and below acromion.
    - Patient Action: internal-external rotation with elbow flexed at $90°$.

- Bony Acoustic Landmark(s): greater tuberosity, bicipital groove, lesser tuberosity, humeral head, and coracoid process.
- Target: long bicipital tendon, subscapularis, subcoracoid recess, and coracoid process. The transducer is moved over the bicipital groove to assess the location of the long head of the biceps brachii tendon in the bicipital groove, with any partial displacement of the tendon from the groove defining subluxation of the tendon, whereas dislocation of the tendon will be seen as a complete medial displacement.
- Scan-Sweep: hover over coracohumeral space.
- Transducer Pressure: feather-touch, so as not to trap subluxing long bicipital tendon or efface subcoracoid bursa/recess.

Superior Shoulder Region

- *Acromioclavicular (AC) joint*
  - Patient Position: seated with hand supinated resting on thigh.
  - Examiner Position: seated, shoulder-to-shoulder with patient.
  - Probe Placement: vertex of shoulder.
  - Bony Acoustic Landmark(s): acromion, joint space, distal clavicle, and anterolateral rim of bony acromion.
  - Target: The superior bony contours of the clavicle and the acromion are well visualized with the bipolar subarticular plates, and the joint space containing fibrocartilage intra-articular disk covered by the joint capsule (Fig. 2.5).
  - Scan-Sweep: lateral rim of acromion to mid-clavicle, then anterior AC joint to scapular spine posteriorly.
  - Transducer Pressure: variable, including feather-touch, so as not to decompress "geyser" sign.
- *Dynamic Exam with Cross-Body Maneuver (only when indicated)*: subluxing or impacting AC joint.

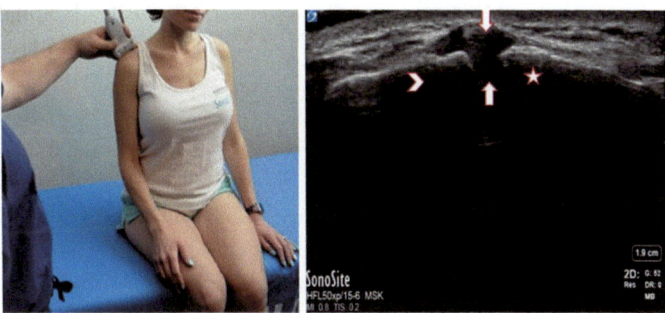

Fig. 2.5 Acromioclavicular (AC) joint. AC joint in Lnx view of transducer placement and corresponding ultrasound image highlighting the joint space (up arrow), clavicle (chevron), acromion (star) and the fibrocartilagenous disc (down arrow)

Anterolateral Shoulder Region

- *Supraspinatus Tendon and Muscle*
  - Patient Position: seated with hand of symptomatic shoulder in hyperextension-internal rotation resting on contralateral scapula (the Dr. Jeffery Cross position).
  - Examiner Position: seated, shoulder-to-shoulder with patient.
  - Probe Placement: radially around the shoulder.
  - Bony Acoustic Landmark(s)

    in long-axis view (*Lnx*): greater tuberosity enthesis, anatomical neck, humeral head subchondral plate, articular hyaline cartilage, acromion, lateral deltoid shelf cortex, and bony bare area.

    in short-axis view (*Sax*): coracoid process, acromion, coracoacromial line, humeral head subchondral plate, lateral deltoid shelf, bony bare area, and the 3 facets of the greater tuberosity with enthesis.

  - Target(s): footprint(s), midsubstances and MTJ of rotator cuff; bursa and articular surface of cuff; subacromialsubdeltoid (SASD) bursa plus synovium; coracoacromial ligament; subacromial space, and deltoid muscle(s).

On Lnx, the supraspinatus parallels the curved contour of the humeral head, and appears as a fibrillar and hyperechoic structure that flattens as it reaches its insertion on the greater tuberosity. Paralleling the tendon superiorly, a thin hyperechoic band is identified as the SASD bursa. From the anterior edge of the supraspinatus tendon, an arbitrary cutoff of 2 cm is used to define the beginning of the infraspinatus tendon (Fig. 2.6a, b).

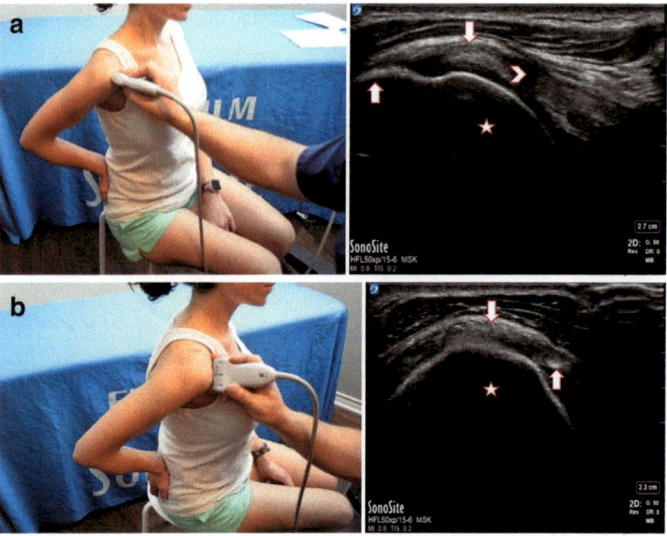

Fig. 2.6 Supraspinatus Tendon and Muscle. Supraspinatus tendon (Sax and Lnx). Lnx view (**a**) and Sax view (**b**) of transducer placement and corresponding ultrasound images. (**a**) Supraspinatus tendon (down arrow), humeral head (star), superior facet (up arrow) are highlighted. The hypoechoic tendon (chevrons) appearance from anisotropy when the tendon is oblique, and should not be confused with a torn tendon. (**b**) Supraspinatus tendon (down arrow), humeral head (star), biceps tendon in rotator interval (up arrow) can be seen

- Scan-Sweep: circumnavigate latitude and longitude of the rotator cuff.
- Transducer Pressure: variable and can be applied to elicit sonographic palpation in order to test for tendinomalacia and unmask tears, and elicit sonographicy palpation.
- *Dynamic Shoulder Evaluation for Subacromial Impingement*
  - Patient Position: seated with arm at side.
  - Examiner Position: seated, shoulder-to-shoulder with patient.
  - Probe Placement:

    For bony arch impingement: bridging acromion to humerus.

    For soft tissue arch impingement: acromioclavicular joint, crossing coracoacromial ligament to humerus.
  - Patient Action: abduction-adduction; with flexion and extension with Neer or Hawkins hand-position; plus supplemental internal-external rotation.
  - Bony Acoustic Landmark(s): Lateral rim of acromion, subacromial space, greater tuberosity, and coracoid process.
  - Target(s): acromial enthesophytes; SASD bursa; supraspinatus and infraspinatus tendons, engaging greater tuberosity; and coracoacromial ligament.
  - Scan-Sweep: hover over subacromial space and rock along with patient's abduction-adduction shoulder motion.

Posterior Shoulder Region

- *Posterior Glenohumeral Joint and Postero-superior Glenoid Labrum*
  - Patient Position: seated with hand supinated resting on thigh.
  - Examiner Position: seated, behind patient.
  - Probe Placement: 2 cm inferior and 1 cm medial to posterolateral corner of acromion (posterior portal of shoulder arthroscopy).
  - Bony Acoustic Landmark(s): glenoid rim and socket, posterior humeral head, and glenohumeral joint line.

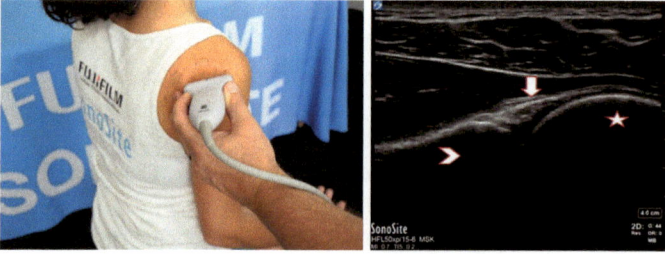

Fig. 2.7 Posterior Glenohumeral Joint and Postero-Superior Glenoid Labrum. Posterior glenohumeral joint and posterosuperior labrum in Lnx view of transducer placement and corresponding ultrasound image. Postero-superior glenoid labrum (down arrow), humeral head (star), and glenoid (chevron) are highlighted

- Target(s): postero-superior glenoid labrum, humeral sub-chondral plate, articular hyaline cartilage, and glenohumeral capsule (Fig. 2.7).
- Scan-Sweep: Upper posterior quadrant of glenohumeral joint.
- *Dynamic exam for ball-and-socket maneuver to locate glenohumeral joint*:
  - Patient Position: seated with hand resting on thigh and elbow at 90° of flexion.
  - Examiner Position: seated, behind patient.
  - Probe Placement: posterior portal of shoulder arthroscopy.
  - Patient Action: internal-external rotation with elbow flexed at 90°.
  - Target(s): glenoid rim, postero-superior glenoid labrum, humeral head, glenohumeral joint, and glenohumeral capsule.
    Supplemental—include bone bare area subjacent to infraspinatus to evaluate for shoulder internal impingement.
  - Scan-Sweep: hover over glenohumeral joint.

- *Spinoglenoid Notch and Spinoglenoid Groove/Glenoid Neck (transit of suprascapular nerve)*
  - Patient Position: seated with hand supinated resting on thigh.
  - Examiner Position: seated, behind patient.
  - Probe Placement: slide medially from glenohumeral joint to base of the scapular spine; spin probe to bridge base of scapular spine with glenoid rim.
  - Bony Acoustic Landmark(s): spinoglenoid groove; spino-glenoid notch and glenoid rim.
  - Target(s): suprascapular neurovascular bundle (Fig. 2.8).
- *Infraspinatus and Teres minor Muscles*
  - Patient Position: seated with hand supinated resting on thigh.
  - Examiner Position: seated, behind patient.
  - Probe Placement: below the scapular spine.
  - Bony Acoustic Landmark(s): base of scapular spine; infraspinatus fossa teres minor fossa; plus posterior and inferior facets of greater tuberosity.
  - Target(s) : muscle volume; fat-muscle composition; infraspinatus and footprint; teres minor and footprint. On Sax, in

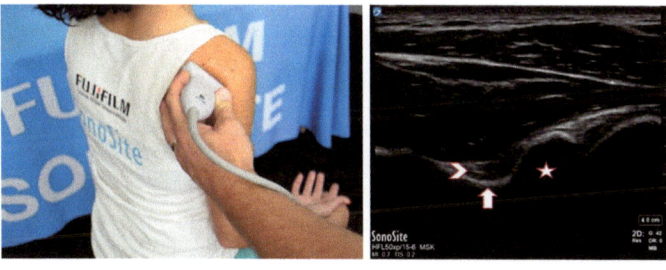

Fig. 2.8 Spinoglenoid Notch and Spinoglenoid Groove. Spinoglenoid notch and groove transducer placement and corresponding ultrasound image. Spinoglenoid notch (up arrow), neurovascular bundle (chevron), and glenoid (star) are highlighted

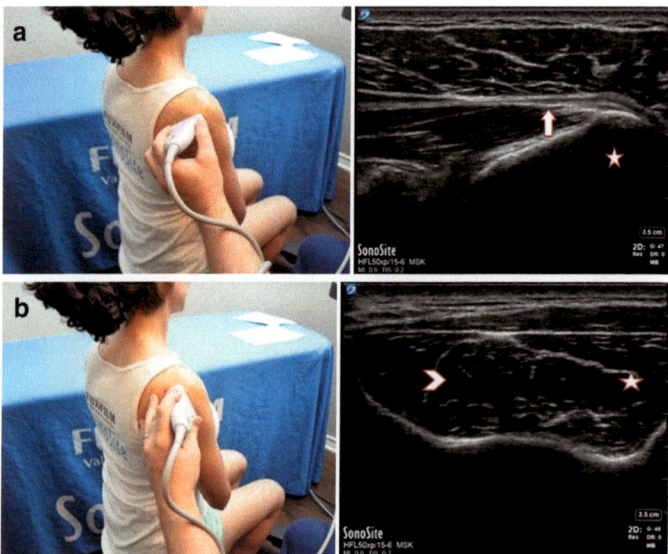

Fig. 2.9 Infraspinatus and Teres minor Muscles and Tendons. Infraspinatus (Sax and Lnx) and teres minor muscles and tendons (Sax). Lnx view (**a**) and Sax view (**b**) of transducer placement and corresponding ultrasound images. (**a**) Infraspinatus tendon (arrow) and humeral head (star) are highlighted. (**b**) Infraspinatus (chevron) and teres minor (star) can be seen

the infraspinous fossa, the infraspinatus and teres minor muscles can be identified deep to the deltoid muscle (Fig. 2.9a, b).
- Scan-Sweep: radially arc over infraspinatus and teres minor muscles.
• *Supraspinatus Muscle*
  - Patient Position: seated with hand supinated resting on thigh.
  - Examiner Position: seated, behind patient.
  - Probe Placement: above scapular spine and medial to bony acromion.

- – Bony Acoustic Landmark(s): (the Y-view of the scapula) superior border of scapular spine with the posterior cortex of clavicle; and supraspinatus fossa.
- – Target(s): muscle volume; fat-muscle composition; supraspinatus muscle and MTJ.
- – Scan-Sweep: radially arc over supraspinatus muscle.
- *Suprascapular Notch*
  - – Patient Position: seated with hand supinated resting on thigh.
  - – Examiner Position: seated, behind patient.
  - – Probe Placement: above scapular spine and medial to bony acromion.
  - – Bony Acoustic Landmark(s): (the Y-view of the scapula) superior border of scapular spine with the posterior cortex of clavicle; supraspinatus fossa; suprascapular notch; and superior glenoid labrum.
  - – Target(s): suprascapular ligament; suprascapular artery above the ligament; suprascapular nerve-vein bundle below the ligament; or suprascapular ganglion when present (Fig. 2.10).

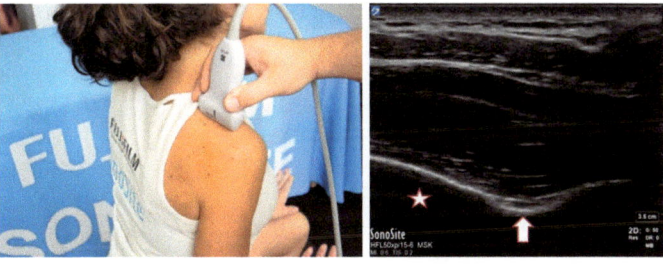

Fig. 2.10 Suprascapular Notch. Suprascapular notch transducer placement and corresponding ultrasound image. Suprascapular notch and neurovascular bundle (up arrow), and scapular spine (star) are highlighted

- *Quadrangular space: Axillary Nerve and Posterior Circumflex Humeral Artery*
  - Patient Position: seated with hand resting on thigh.
  - Examiner Position: seated, behind patient.
  - Probe Placement: inferior to the posterior portal of shoulder arthroscopy, parallel to the shaft of the humerus.
  - Bony Acoustic Landmark(s): humerus, lateral border of scapula.
  - Target: The quadrangular space can be identified between the teres minor, teres major, long head of the triceps brachii, and the humerus. The axillary nerve and posterior circumflex humeral artery can be identified in the space.

Ultrasound of the Elbow

3

- Transducer: Linear-array.
- Apply variable pressure with transducer, from feather-touch to 10 lbs pressure.
- Doppler deployed for all blood vessels, and suspected lesions.

Anterior Elbow Region

- *Biceps brachii muscle, Brachialis muscle, Brachial artery and vein, Median nerve*
  - Patient Position: seated with elbow neutral on table and hand supinated, pillow can be placed under elbow joint to maximize extension.
  - Examiner Position: seated facing the patient.
  - Probe Placement: antecubital crease.
  - Bony Acoustic Landmark(s): distal humeral articular surface.
  - Target: Superficial biceps and deeper larger brachialis muscles can be found in supracondylar region anterior to the humerus, between the brachioradialis laterally and pronator teres medially, and traced distally along their tendons. The muscles appear as hypoechoic fascicles with intervening hyperechoic fibroadipose septa. Medial to the muscles, the brachial artery and vein, alongside the median nerve can be

© The Author(s), under exclusive license to Springer Nature Switzerland AG 2022
M. M. El-Othmani et al., *Sports Medicine and Musculoskeletal Ultrasound*, https://doi.org/10.1007/978-3-031-11764-0_3

found (nerve medial to artery). The median nerve will have a speckled fascicular appearance on Sax.
- Scan-Sweep: 5 cm above and 5 cm below the ulnohumeral joint, and sweeping medially to laterally.
- *Distal Biceps and Brachialis tendons including dynamic scanning*
  - Patient Position: seated with elbow neutral on table and hand supinated, pillow can be placed under elbow joint to maximize extension.
  - Examiner Position: seated facing the patient.
  - Probe Placement: antecubital crease.
  - Bony Acoustic Landmark(s): capitellum, radial head, radial tuberosity, coronoid process.
  - Target: Distal biceps tendon has an oblique course from surface to depth, and portions may appear hypoechoic if the probe is not maintained parallel to it. Probe in Lnx of the tendon and distal portion gently pushed against the arm to ensure parallelism. At the myotendinous junction, the lacertus fibrosus is identified as an aponeurotic flattening extending to the medial deep fascia of the forearm and covering the median nerve and brachial artery (Fig. 3.1).
  - Scan-Sweep: from muscle bellies identified earlier to the radial tuberosity (biceps tendon) and coronoid process (brachialis tendon).

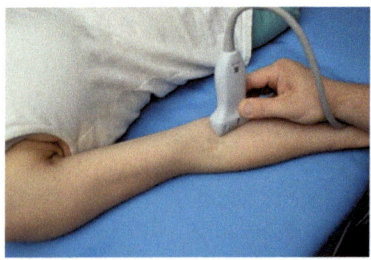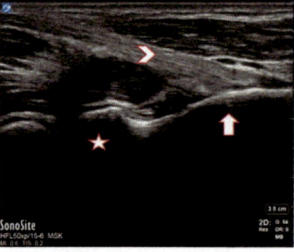

Fig. 3.1 Distal Biceps and Brachialis tendons. Distal biceps brachii tendon in Lnx view, images of transducer placement and corresponding ultrasound findings. Biceps tendon (chevron), radial head (star) and the insertion at the tuberosity (up arrow) can be seen

- *Anterior Humeroradial and Humeroulnar joint*
  - Patient Position: seated with elbow neutral on table and hand supinated, pillow can be placed under elbow joint to maximize extension.
  - Examiner Position: seated facing the patient.
  - Bony Acoustic Landmark(s): capitellum, trochlea, radial head, radial fossa, coronoid fossa, coronoid recess.
  - Probe Placement: perpendicular to humerus for Sax images and parallel to it for Lnx images.
  - Target: Sax images over the distal humeral extremity demonstrate wavy osteochondral surface of the convex capitellum and of the concave trochlea (articular cartilage appears as a uniform hypoechoic band overlying the subchondral bone). Lnx images over the radiocapitellar joint are useful to study the radial fossa with the radial recess, and the coronoid fossa with its respective coronoid recess. The radiocapitellar joint is located laterally and the trochlea-ulna joint is found medially (Fig. 3.2a, b). The anterior fat pads are evaluated superficially to the recesses.
- *Radial and Posterior Interosseous Nerves*
  - Patient Position: seated with elbow neutral on table and hand supinated, pillow can be placed under elbow joint to maximize extension.
  - Examiner Position: seated facing the patient.
  - Probe Placement: anterolateral elbow, perpendicular to joint line.
  - Bony Acoustic Landmark(s): capitellum, radial head.
  - Target: At the proximal elbow level, and in Sax, find the radial nerve proximal to the joint between the brachioradialis and the brachialis muscles (Fig. 3.3a). The nerve can be followed distally to its bifurcation into the superficial sensory branch and the posterior interosseous nerve as it pierces the supinator muscle after coursing through the radial tunnel (Fig. 3.3b).
  - Scan-Sweep: 5 cm above and 5 cm below the radiohumeral joint.
- *Dynamic scanning of annular recess of the neck of the radius (supination/pronation)*

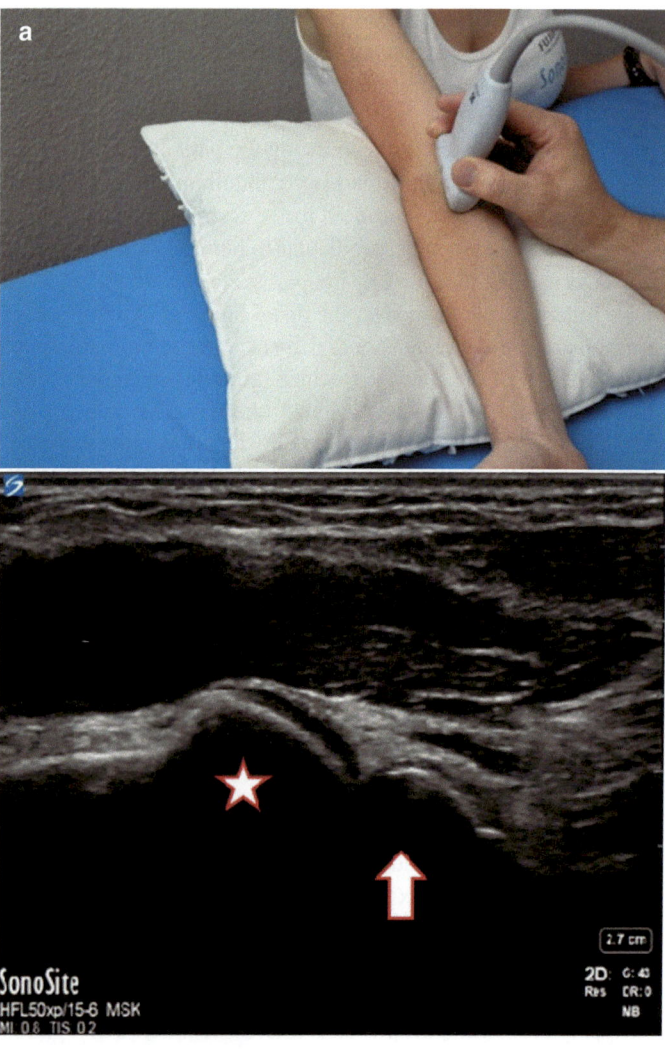

Fig. 3.2 Anterior humeroradial and humeroulnar joint. Anterior humeroradial and humeroulnar joints transducer placement and corresponding ultrasound images. The transducer should be moved medially and laterally from
the pictured position for improved joint visualization (**a**) Humerus trochlea
(star) and proximal ulna (arrow) are highlighted. (**b**) Humerus capitellum
(star) and radial head (arrow) can be seen

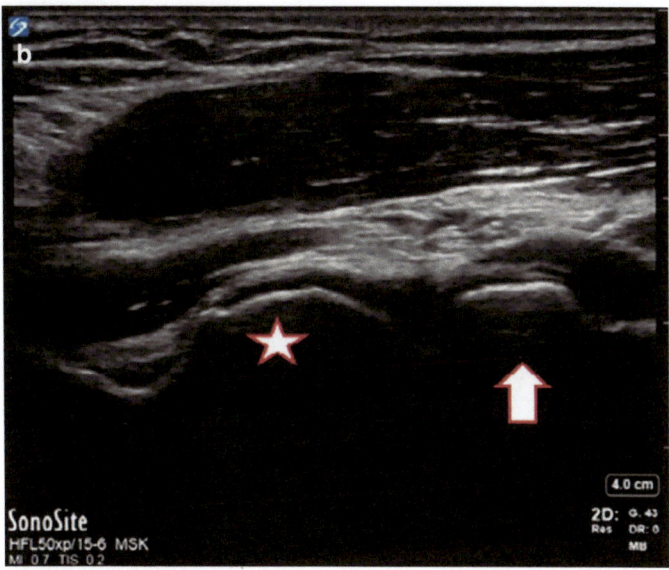

Fig. 3.2 (continued)

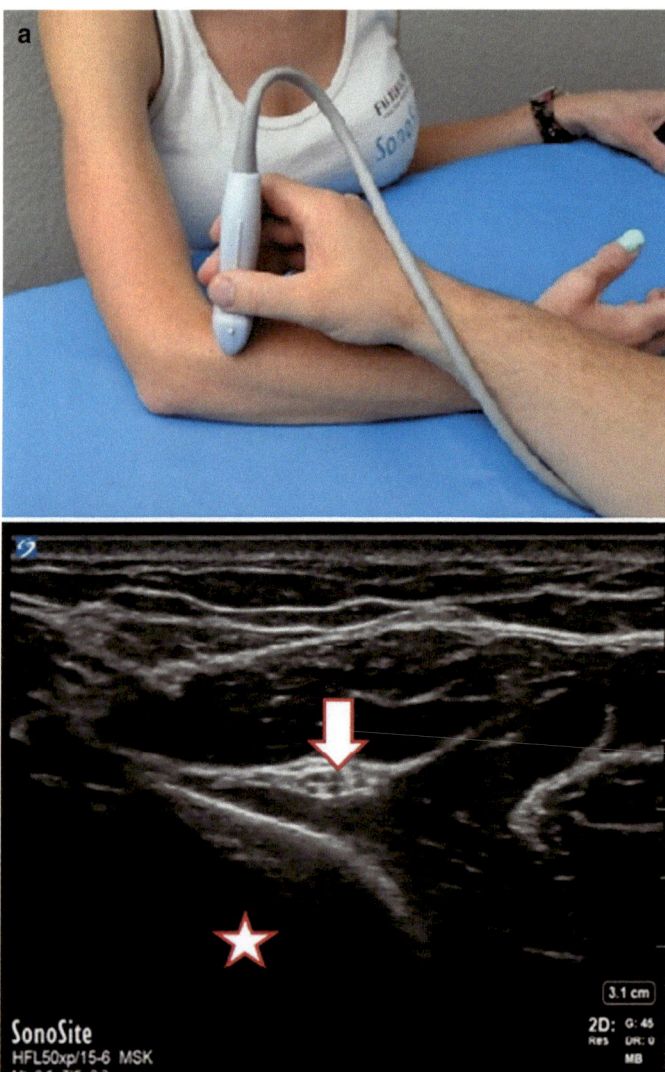

Fig. 3.3 Radial and Posterior Interosseous Nerves (PIN). Radial nerve in Sax view with transducer placement and corresponding ultrasound images. The transducer is moved proximally and distally to highlight (**a**) Radial nerve (down arrow) and humerus (star) prior to bifurcation proximally and (**b**) PIN (down arrow) and superficial sensory branch (up arrow) distally at the level of the radial head

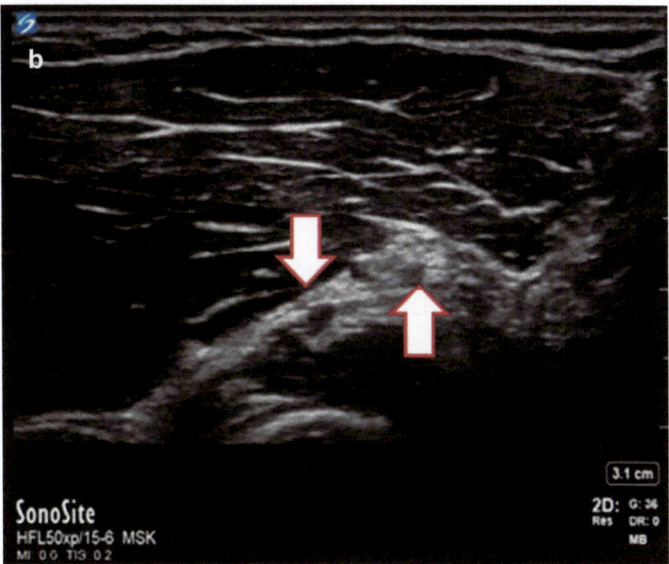

Fig. 3.3 (continued)

Notes

1. Target structures are scanned proximal and distal as clinically indicated.
2. Multiple views of the distal biceps are possible, including:
   a. Anterior approach
   b. Medial (pronator window)
   c. Lateral
   d. Posterior (via interosseous space)

Lateral Elbow Region

- *Proximal attachment of Brachioradialis and Extensor carpi radialis longus*
  - Patient Position: seated with elbow in extension with thumb up or with elbow at 90 degrees of flexion.
  - Examiner Position: seated to the side of the patient.
  - Probe Placement: parallel to the humerus.

- Bony Acoustic Landmark(s): lateral epicondyle.
- Target: Lateral epicondyle appears as smooth down-sloping hyperechoic structure.
- *Common extensor tendon origin (CETO) and muscles*
  - Patient Position: seated with hand pronated and with elbow at 90 degrees of flexion.
  - Examiner Position: seated to the side of the patient.
  - Probe Placement: parallel to the humerus for a Lnx view and perpendicular to it for a Sax view.
  - Bony Acoustic Landmark(s): lateral epicondyle, radial head.
  - Target: The CETO between the subcutaneous tissue and the radial collateral ligament appears as a beak-shaped hyperechoic origin on Lnx. The extensor carpi radialis brevis is the deepest, and the extensor digitorum is the most superficial (Fig. 3.4).
- *Lateral collateral ligament complex*
  - Patient Position: seated with hand pronated and with elbow at 90 degrees of flexion.
  - Examiner Position: seated to the side of the patient.
  - Probe Placement: parallel to the humerus for a Lnx view and perpendicular to it for a Sax view.

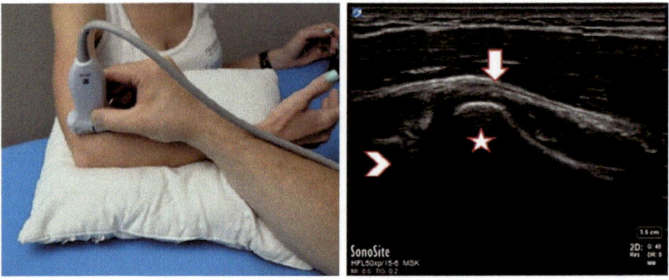

Fig. 3.4 Common extensor tendon origin (CETO) and muscles. CETO Lnx view of transducer placement and corresponding ultrasound image. The lateral epicondyle (chevron), and radial head (star) are highlighted

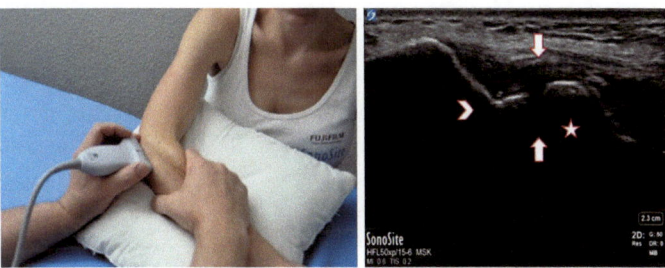

Fig. 3.5 Lateral collateral ligament (LCL) complex and lateral radiocapitellar joint. Lateral collateral ligament complex (Lnx view) transducer placement and corresponding ultrasound image. LCL (down arrow), humerus (chevron), radial head (star), and radiocapitellar joint space (up arrow) are highlighted

- Bony Acoustic Landmark(s): lateral epicondyle, radial head.
- Target: The CETO is separated from the joint capsule by the lateral collateral ligamentous complex, including the annular ligament, the radial collateral ligament, and the lateral ulnar collateral ligament (LUCL) relative to the common extensor tendon origin (Fig. 3.5). To evaluate the lateral ulnar collateral ligament, the elbow should be with the hand supinated and pronated applying a varus stress to stress the ligament.
- *Humeroradial joint (including dynamic imaging as indicated)*
  - Patient Position: seated with hand pronated and with elbow at 90 degrees of flexion.
  - Examiner Position: seated to the side of the patient.
  - Probe Placement: perpendicular to the humerus.
  - Bony Acoustic Landmark(s): capitellum, radial head.
  - Target: A lateral synovial fringe that fills the superficial portion of the lateral aspect of the radiocapitellar joint can be appreciated on Lnx. This meniscoid-like structure may become enlarged and produce pain and/or mechanical symptoms, at which time it is referred to as a plica.

- Dynamic scanning during passive pronation and supination of the forearm may help to assess the status of the radial head and annular ligament.
- *Radial nerve bifurcation and course through supinator muscle*
  - Similar landmarks and approach as in anterior elbow region.
  - Radial nerve divides distally into superficial cutaneous sensory branch and the posterior interosseous nerve. The posterior interosseous nerve can be visualized as it pierces the supinator muscle and enters the arcade of Frohse, passing between the superficial and deep parts.

Medial Elbow Region

- *Medial epicondyle, common flexor-pronator tendon and muscles*
  - Patient Position: Leaning towards the examined side with the forearm in forceful external rotation while keeping the elbow extended or slightly flexed.
  - Examiner Position: seated at patient's side.
  - Probe Placement: parallel to ulna shaft.
  - Bony Acoustic Landmark(s): medial epicondyle, ulna.
  - Target: Probe placed over the medial epicondyle reveals the common flexor tendon in its Lnx (Fig. 3.6). The tendon is

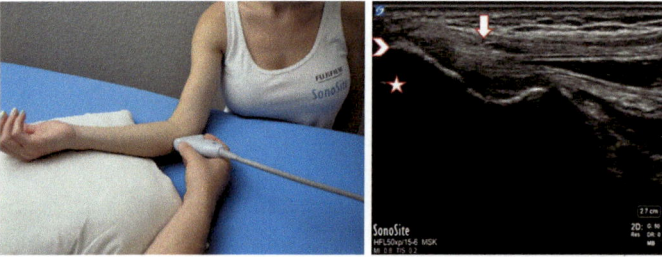

Fig. 3.6 Medial epicondyle, common flexor-pronator tendon and muscles. Common flexor-pronator tendon in Lnx view of transducer placement and corresponding ultrasound image. The medial epicondyle (star), the common tendon (arrow) and its insertion (chevron) are highlighted

shorter and larger than the CETO. Deep to this tendon, the anterior bundle of the medial collateral ligament can be assessed.

- *Medial Antebrachial cutaneous nerve (MABC)*
    - Patient Position: Leaning towards the examined side with the forearm in forceful external rotation while keeping the elbow extended or slightly flexed.
    - Examiner Position: seated at patient's side.
    - Probe Placement: parallel to ulna shaft.
    - Bony Acoustic Landmark(s): medial epicondyle, ulna.
    - Target: The MABC nerve can be identified along the basilic vein in the subcutaneous layer between the brachialis and the triceps brachii muscles.
- *Humeroulnar joint*
- Patient Position: Leaning towards the examined side with the forearm in forceful external rotation while keeping the elbow extended or slightly flexed.
    - Examiner Position: seated at patient's side.
    - Probe Placement: perpendicular to humerus for Sax images and parallel to it for Lnx images.
    - Bony Acoustic Landmark(s): Trochlea, ulna.
    - Target: At the ulnotrochlear joint, the hyaline cartilage appears as a thin hypoechoic band superficial to the hyperechoic cortex and deep to the hyperechoic joint capsule. On Lnx view, a hyperechoic anterior fat pad can be identified within the coronoid fossa. The trochlea would appear as a V-shaped structure on Sax.
- *Ulnar collateral ligament and Dynamic valgus stress of ulnar collateral ligament (as indicated)*
    - Patient Position: seating upright or supine with the shoulder abducted and externally rotated and the elbow in 90° of flexion.
    - Probe Placement: parallel to ulnar shaft.
    - Bony Acoustic Landmark(s): medial epicondyle, ulna.
    - Target: anterior band of the medial collateral ligament is depicted as tense fibrillar structure crossing the trochlea-ulna joint with elbow in flexion (Fig. 3.7a).
    - Valgus stress for UCL incompetence (Fig. 3.7b).

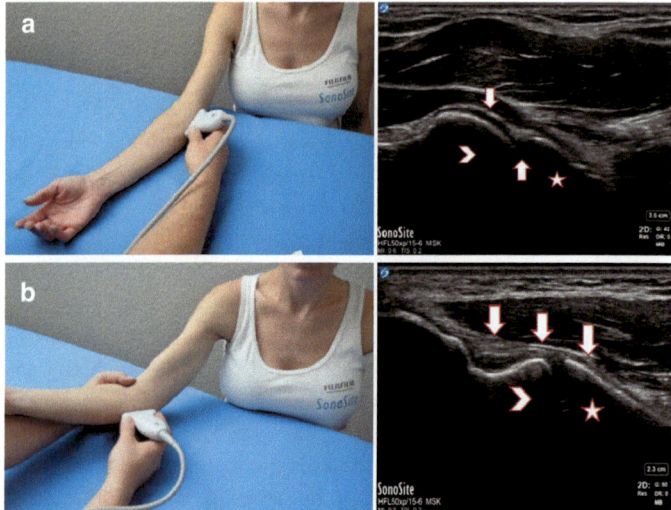

Fig. 3.7 Humeroulnar joint and Ulnar collateral ligament (UCL). Transducer placement and corresponding ultrasound images for Humeroulnar joint assessment (**a**) and stress evaluation of the UCL (**b**). (**a**) Joint space (up arrow), ulnar collateral ligament (down arrow), ulna (star), and trochlea (chevron) can be seen. (**b**) Ulnar collateral ligament (down arrows) can be better visualized following valgus stress application at a slightly flexed elbow

- *Dynamic flexion-extension (as indicated)*
  - Evaluate for ulnar nerve subluxation (Fig. 3.8a, b).
  - Evaluate for snapping triceps tendon.

Notes
1. Static examination of the ulnar nerve is facilitated by placing the elbow in an extended position, whereas dynamic testing requires elbow flexion.
2. Evaluation for ulnar nerve subluxation and snapping triceps may include passive flexion, active flexion, and/or resisted extension from a fully flexed position.

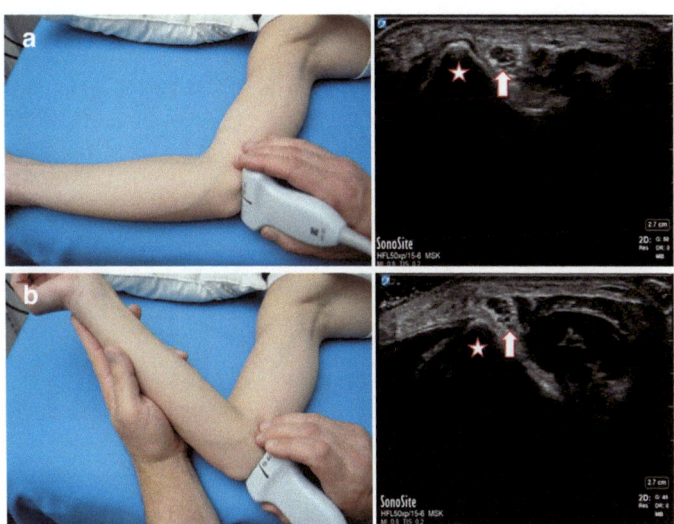

Fig. 3.8 Dynamic ulnar nerve assessment. Ulnar nerve in Sax view with elbow in flexion (**a**) and increased flexion (**b**) with transducer placement and corresponding ultrasound images. (**a**) Ulnar nerve (arrow) and medial epicondyle (star) are highlighted. (**b**) Anterior translation of ulnar nerve within the cubital tunnel following increased flexion can be seen

Posterior Elbow Region

- *Triceps muscle, tendon, Olecranon process, fossa, bursa, and posterior joint space*
  - Patient Position: In crab position—elbow flexed to 90 degrees and palm resting on the table. Alternatively, patient's pronated hand slides cranio-caudally from waistline to knee.
  - Examiner Position: seated by patient's side.
  - Probe Placement: parallel to humeral shaft.
  - Bony Acoustic Landmark(s): Olecranon.
  - Target: Evaluate triceps muscle and tendon, on Lnx and Sax, proximal to the olecranon insertion. Deep to the tri-

ceps, the olecranon fossa and the posterior olecranon can be evaluated. At 45° of flexion, intra-articular fluid tends to move from the anterior synovial space to the olecranon recess, allowing identification of small effusions. Feather-touch probe pressure should be applied when examining the olecranon bursa (Fig. 3.9a, b).

- *Ulnar nerve (also included in medial region scan)*
  - Patient Position: elbow may be fully extended and the arm internally rotated to avoid compression of the ulnar nerve at the cubital tunnel.
  - Examiner Position: seated facing patient's olecranon.
  - Probe Placement: parallel to arm and forearm.
  - Bony Acoustic Landmarks: Olecranon, medial epicondyle.

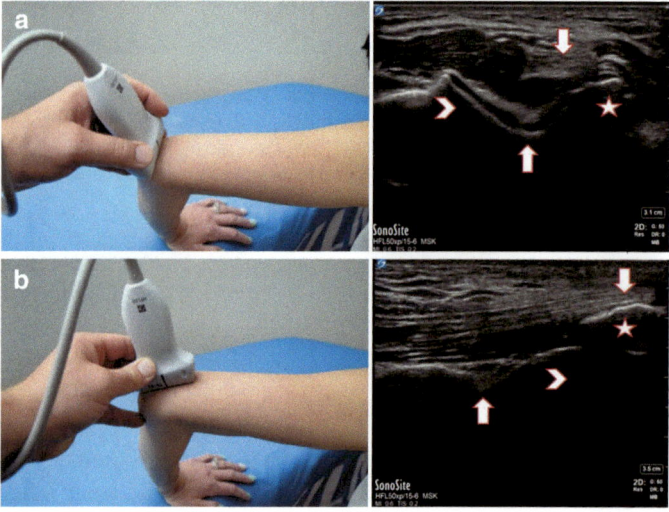

Fig. 3.9 Triceps muscle and tendon, Olecranon process, fossa, bursa, and posterior joint space. Triceps tendon (Sax and Lnx). Sax view (**a**) and Lnx view (**b**) of transducer placement and corresponding ultrasound images. Olecranon (star), Trochlea (chevron), Triceps tendon (down arrow), and Olecranon fossa (up arrow) are highlighted

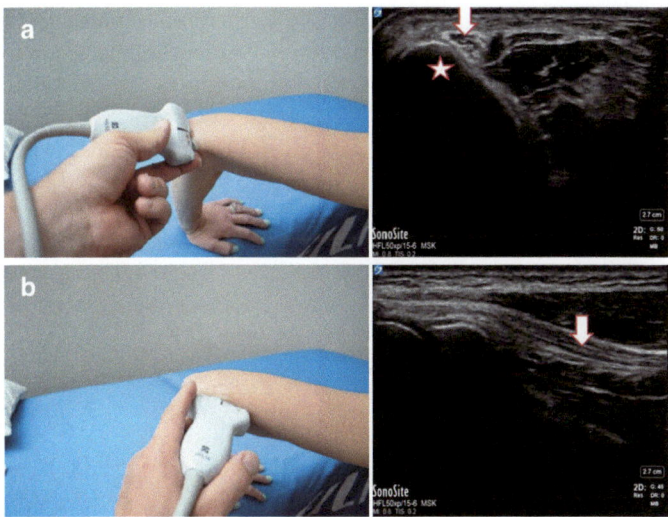

Fig. 3.10 Ulnar nerve (also included in medial region scan). Ulnar nerve (Sax and Lnx). Sax view (**a**) and Lnx view (**b**) of transducer placement and corresponding ultrasound images. Ulnar nerve (arrow) and medial epicondyle (star) are highlighted

- Target: Assess the ulnar nerve in the cubital tunnel at the medial side of the elbow under the Osborne ligament (Fig. 3.10a, b).
- *Dynamic flexion-extension (as indicated) (also included in medial region scan)*
  - evaluate for ulnar nerve subluxation.
  - evaluate for snapping triceps tendon.
- *Radial and Posterior Antebrachial Cutaneous nerves (PABC)*
  - Patient Position: In crab position—elbow flexed to 90 degrees and palm resting on the table. Alternatively, patient's pronated hand slides cranio-caudally from waist-line to knee.
  - Examiner Position: seated by patient's side.
  - Probe Placement: parallel to humeral shaft, at the posterior mid-arm level.

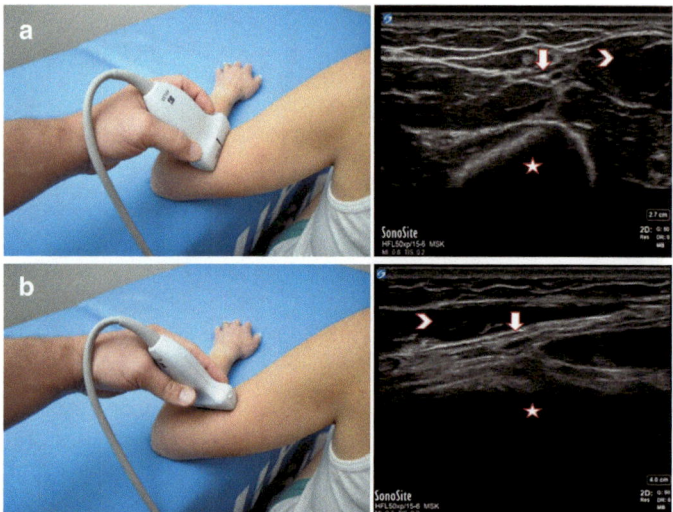

Fig. 3.11 Posterior antebrachial cutaneous nerves (PABC). Posterior ante-brachial butaneous nerve (Sax and Lnx). Sax view (**a**) and Lnx view (**b**) of transducer placement and corresponding ultrasound images. PABC (arrow), lateral epicondyle (star), and lateral triceps (chevron) are highlighted

- Bony Acoustic Landmark(s): Distal humerus, Olecranon.
- Target: The radial nerve can be identified after exiting the spiral groove, underneath the lateral head of the triceps bra-chii. The PABC nerve can be seen as it branches from the radial nerve and followed as it emerges in the subcutaneous layer (Fig. 3.11a, b).

Notes
1. Static examination of the ulnar nerve is facilitated by placing the elbow in an extended position, whereas dynamic testing requires elbow flexion.
2. Evaluation for ulnar nerve subluxation and snapping triceps may include passive flexion, active flexion, and/or resisted extension from a fully flexed position.

Ultrasound of the Wrist and Hand

4

- Transducer(s): Linear-array and/or compact linear-array (e.g., "hockey stick")
- Variable applied pressure with transducer.

Volar Wrist and Hand Region

- **Carpal tunnel and its contents (Median Nerve (MN), Flexor Digitorum Superficialis (FDS) and Profundus (FDP), and Flexor Pollicis Longus (FPL))**
  - Patient Position: seated with both hand(s) supinated resting on table.
  - Examiner Position: seated in front of the patient.
  - Probe Placement
    Proximal: just distal to palmar crease, in Sax initially to identify bony acoustic landmarks.
    Distal: in Sax initially to identify bony acoustic landmarks of the distal carpal tunnel.
  - Bony Acoustic Landmark(s)
    Proximal: scaphoid tubercle (radial) and pisiform (ulnar).
    Distal: trapezium tubercle (radial) and hook of the hamate (ulnar).

© The Author(s), under exclusive license to Springer Nature Switzerland AG 2022
M. M. El-Othmani et al., *Sports Medicine and Musculoskeletal Ultrasound*, https://doi.org/10.1007/978-3-031-11764-0_4

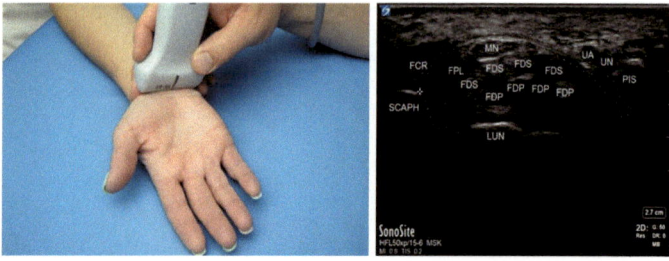

Fig. 4.1 Carpal tunnel and its contents—Median Nerve (MN), Flexor Digitorum Superficialis (FDS) and Profundus (FDP), and Flexor Pollicis Longus (FPL). Carpal tunnel and its content Sax view of transducer placement and corresponding ultrasound image. The scaphoid, lunate, and pisiform bones, ulnar artery (UA) and nerve (UN), flexor carpi radialis (FCR), and the content of the carpal tunnel are highlighted

- Target: The transverse ligament forms the roof of the carpal tunnel and runs from scaphoid to pisiform. The nine flexor tendons can be seen underneath the transverse ligament. The four tendons from the FDS will be the most superficial, and the four from the FDP will be deeper. The most radial tendon in the tunnel will be the FPL. Slightly radial and superficial, the median nerve can be seen as an elliptical structure with the typical "honey comb" echo-signature (Fig. 4.1).
- Dynamic examination: the respective tendons within the carpal tunnel can be verified with flexion and extension of the respective fingers and assessment of tendon and MN motion.
- Scan-sweep: Sweep the transducer up and down over the median nerve to complete a systematic examination in its short axis from the distal radius through the palm (beyond the distal edge of the transverse ligament).
- **Flexor Carpi Radialis tendon and Radial artery**
  - Patient Position: seated with both hand(s) supinated resting on table.
  - Examiner Position: seated in front of the patient.

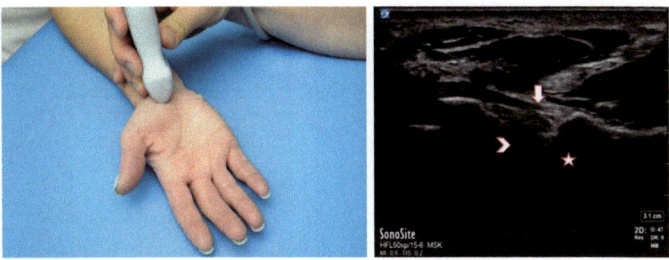

Fig. 4.2 Flexor carpi radialis tendon and radial artery. FCR tendon Lnx view of transducer placement and corresponding ultrasound images. FCR tendon (arrow), radius (chevron), and scaphoid (star) are highlighted

- – Probe Placement for FCR: over palmar crease, radial side.
- – Bony Acoustic Landmark(s): scaphoid tubercle.
- – Target: The FCR tendon can be tracked distally across the scaphoid tubercle to its insertion into the second metacarpal (Fig. 4.2).
- **Ulnar nerve and Ulnar artery in Guyon's canal**
  - – Patient Position: seated with both hand(s) supinated resting on table.
  - – Examiner Position: seated in front of the patient.
  - – Probe Placement: over palmar crease, ulnar side.
  - – Bony Acoustic Landmark(s): pisiform.
  - – Target: Identify the ulnar artery (radial) and nerve (ulnar) between the transverse ligament and accessory ligament, and follow the nerve distally on Sax to examine its two branches: the superficial sensory branch and the deep motor branch (coursing alongside the hook of hamate) (Fig. 4.3).
- **Flexor Carpi Ulnaris tendon**
  - – Patient Position: seated with both hand(s) supinated resting on table.
  - – Examiner Position: seated in front of the patient.
  - – Probe Placement: over palmar crease, ulnar side.
  - – Bony Acoustic Landmark(s): pisiform, hook of the hamate and base of fifth metacarpal.

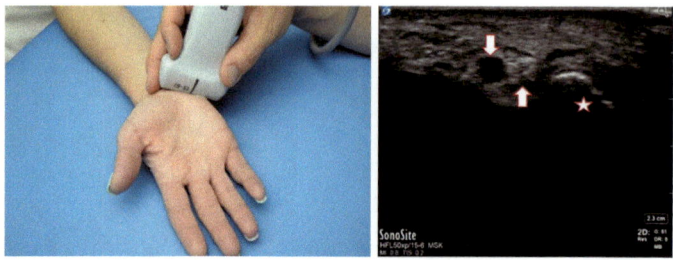

Fig. 4.3 Ulnar nerve and ulnar artery in Guyon's canal. Ulnar nerve and artery Sax view of transducer placement and corresponding ultrasound images. Ulnar nerve (up arrow), ulnar artery (down arrow), and pisiform (star) are highlighted

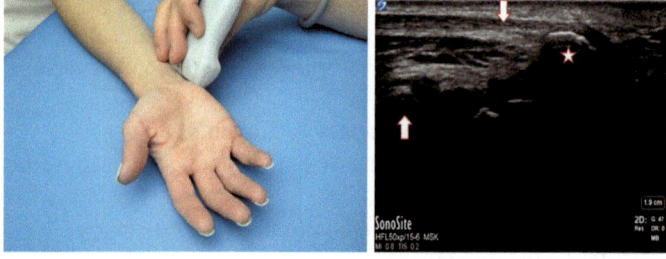

Fig. 4.4 Flexor carpi ulnaris (FCU) tendon. FCU tendon Lnx view of transducer placement and corresponding ultrasound images. FCU tendon (down arrow), ulna (up arrow), and pisiform (star) are highlighted

- – Target: The FCU tendon can be identified at its three insertion(s) on the pisiform-hook-metacarpal, then tracked proximally on Sax for complete assessment (Fig. 4.4).
- **Finger A1 Pulley (Trigger Finger assessment)**
  - – Patient Position: seated with hand in supination.
  - – Examiner Position: seated in front of the patient.
  - – Probe Placement: Orthogonal plane(s) over the distal palmar crease (level of MCP joint) at the level of the finger of interest
  - – Bony Acoustic Landmark(s): MCP joint and FDS plus FDP.

- Target: The A1 pulley can be identified on the volar aspect at the level of the MCP. Trigger finger is assessed by the presence of a diffuse hypoechoic thickening of the A1 pulley and underlying flexor tendon swelling and rounder appearance in Sax views under the thickened pulley, with fluid collection in the flexor sheath (suggestive of tenosynovitis) (Fig. 4.5a, b).
- Dynamic examination: The finger of interest is moved in flexion and extension and the locking and snapping of the flexor tendon at the MCP level can be visualized.
- **Finger A2 and A4 Pulleys (Bowstring Lesion assessment)**
  - Patient Position: seated with hand in supination.
  - Examiner Position: seated in front of the patient.

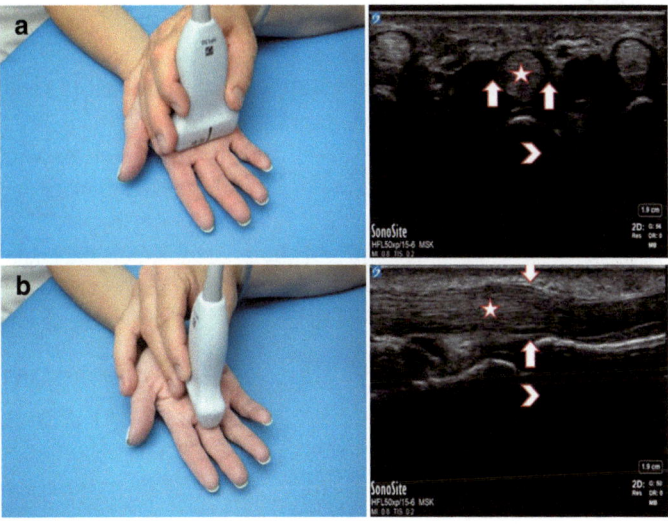

Fig. 4.5 Fingers A1 pulley system. Fingers pulley system, A1 pulley at the metacarpal joint (Sax and Lnx). Lnx view (**a**) and Sax view (**b**) of transducer placement and corresponding ultrasound images. (**a**) A1 pulley (up arrow), flexor tendon (star), and metacarpal head (chevron) are highlighted. (**b**) A1 pulley (up and down arrows), flexor tendon (star), and MCP joint (chevron) can be seen

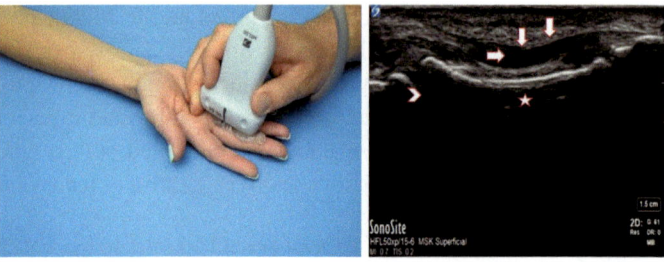

Fig. 4.6 Fingers A2 pulley system. The A2 pulley system Sax view of transducer placement and corresponding ultrasound images. The A2 pulley (down arrows) can be seen around the flexor tendon (horizontal arrow) as it runs over the proximal phalanx (star). The MCP joint (chevron) is highlighted, and the palmar plate can be seen at the level of the joint between the tendon and underlying bone

- – Probe Placement: Orthogonal plane(s) over the diaphysis of proximal phalanx of the finger of interest.
- – Bony Acoustic Landmark(s): PIP joint, proximal phalanx (PP), DIP joint, middle phalanx (MP), and A2 pulley.
- – Target: A2 pulley is assessed over the middle-to-distal of PP. In normal examination it is identified as the thickest and longest annular pulley, and is seen as a linear hyperechoic or hypoechoic thickening of the tendon sheath on a Lnx scan (Fig. 4.6). The A4 pulley can be identified over the MP near the DIP joint. The presence of edema within the pulley or disruption of its fibers is indicative of tear.
- – Dynamic examination: The finger of interest is moved in flexion against resistance and bowstringing of the flexor tendons at the corresponding injury site can be observed.
- – Scan-sweep: from the PP to the DIP to assess all pulleys (most notably A2 and A4).
- • **Palmar plate**
  - – Patient Position: seated with hand in supination.
  - – Examiner Position: seated in front of the patient.
  - – Probe Placement: Transverse plane over the palmar plate of the finger of interest at the proximal interphalangeal (PIP) joint.

- Bony Acoustic Landmark(s): PIP joint, and FDP.
- Target: A hypoechoic cleft within a swollen volar plate is indicative of a rupture of the plate. Volar plate is assessed for any gaps or bony attachments.
- **Flexor Digitorum Profundus (Jersey finger assessment)**
  - Patient Position: seated with hand in supination.
  - Examiner Position: seated in front of the patient.
  - Probe Placement: Orthogonal plane(s) over the distal phalanx and the DIP joint of the finger of interest.
  - Bony Acoustic Landmark(s): DIP joint, distal phalanx (DP), and FDS.
  - Target: In normal fingers, the FDP can be traced to its insertion at the base of the DP. In partial tears of the tendon, a hypoechoic, fusiform swelling and focal discontinuity of the internal fibrillar appearance will be seen. In complete tears, the tendon can't be identified at its insertion site, and the end of the frayed retracted tendon presents as an irregular and hypoechoic lesion. In cases of bony avulsion, the piece of bone attached to the retracted FDP can be identified (Fig. 4.7).
  - Dynamic examination: Should be routinely performed during active and passive motion and contraction against resistance to assess continuity of the tendon and to identify partial tears.

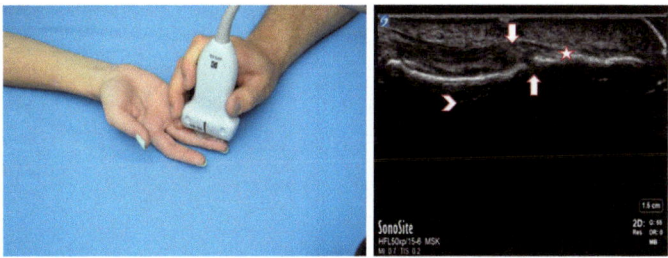

Fig. 4.7 Flexor Digitorum Profundus (FDP) insertion at distal phalanx (DP) Jersey finger. FDP tendon at DP insertion Lnx view of transducer placement and corresponding ultrasound images. FDP tendon (down arrow) can be seen as it inserts on the DP (star). The underlying distal interphalangeal joint (up arrow) and middle phalanx (chevron) are highlighted

Notes

1. All tendons may be traced proximally or distally as clinically indicated.
2. During dynamic finger flexion-extension, both the median nerve and flexor tendons demonstrate longitudinal excursion, although the nerve translates less than the tendons.
3. The region of the flexor carpi radialis and radial artery should be closely examined for the presence of an occult volar wrist ganglion.

Ulnar/Medial Wrist Region

- **Extensor Carpi Ulnaris (ECU) tendon and muscle, and Triangular Fibrocartilage Complex (TFCC)**
  - Patient Position: seated with hand in slight dorsiflexion and radial deviation resting on table.
  - Examiner Position: seated in front of the patient.
  - Probe Placement: base of the hypothenar.
  - Bony Acoustic Landmark(s): ulnar groove, ulnar styloid, DRUJ, and triquetrum.
  - Target: The ECU is identified between the ulnar head and styloid process, and then followed on Sax and Lnx planes. At the ulnar styloid, the gap between the styloid and the radius is filled with the TFCC (Fig. 4.8).

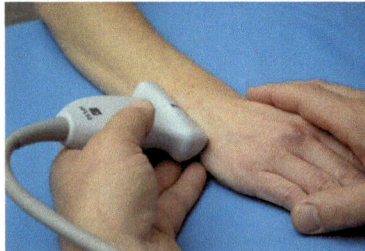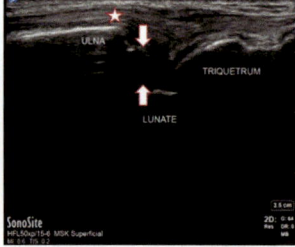

Fig. 4.8 Extensor Carpi Ulnaris (ECU) tendon and muscle, and Triangular Fibrocartilage Complex (TFCC). ECU tendon and TFCC Lnx view of transducer placement and corresponding ultrasound images. TFCC (arrows) and ECU (star) are highlighted

– Dynamic examination: The ECU is assessed for instability through wrist pronation-supination. The tendon typically becomes unstable in supination.

Radial/Lateral Wrist Region

- **Radial Artery, Vein, and Nerve**
  - Patient Position: seated with hand in neutral pronation-supination with ulnar side resting on table.
  - Examiner Position: seated in front of the patient.
  - Probe Placement: Orthogonal plane(s) over the radial side of the wrist, proximal to radial styloid.
  - Bony Acoustic Landmark(s): radius and scaphoid.
  - Target: The radial artery is deep and the sensory nerve is superficial to the first compartment (Fig. 4.9).
- **Extensor Retinaculum, First dorsal compartments (Abductor Pollicis Longus, Extensor Pollicis Brevis)**
  - Patient Position: seated with hand in neutral pronation-supination with ulnar side resting on table.
  - Examiner Position: seated in front of the patient.
  - Probe Placement: Transverse plane over the radial side of the wrist.

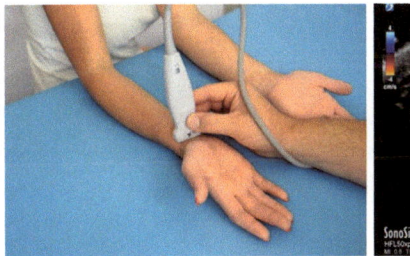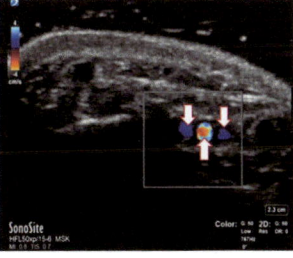

Fig. 4.9 Radial artery and veins. Radial artery and nerve at the wrist level. Sax view of transducer placement and corresponding ultrasound images. Radial artery (up arrow) and radial veins (down arrows) are highlighted using the Doppler function

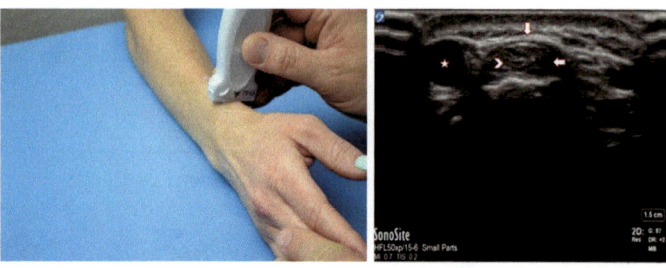

Fig. 4.10 Extensor retinaculum, First dorsal compartments (Abductor Pollicis Longus (APL), Extensor Pollicis Brevis (EPB)). First dorsal compartment Sax view of transducer placement and corresponding ultrasound images. APL (horizontal arrow) and EPB (chevron) in first dorsal compartment with overlying extensor retinaculum (down arrow) and cephalic vein (star) are highlighted

- Bony Acoustic Landmark(s): radial styloid.
- Target: The APL (ventral) and EPB (dorsal) are identified and then followed on Sax plane down to the distal insertion (Fig. 4.10).

Dorsal Wrist and Hand Region

- **Extensor Retinaculum, Second dorsal compartments (Extensor Carpi Radialis Longus and Extensor Carpi Radialis Brevis)**
  - Patient Position: seated with hand in pronation with palm resting on table.
  - Examiner Position: seated in front of the patient.
  - Probe Placement: Transverse plane over the radial side of the wrist.
  - Bony Acoustic Landmark(s): radial styloid, Lister's tubercle.
  - Target: The ECRL (radial) and ECRB (ulnar) are identified and then followed on Sax plane as they run deep to tendons of first compartment (Fig. 4.11).

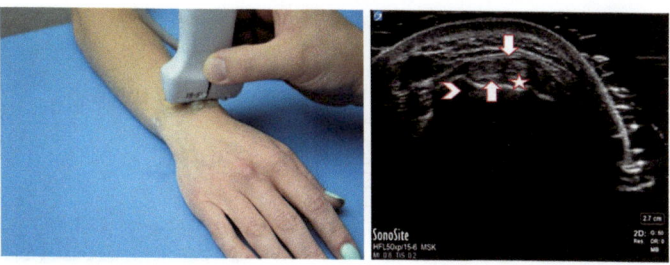

Fig. 4.11 Extensor retinaculum, second dorsal compartments (Extensor Carpi Radialis Longus (ECRL) and Extensor Carpi Radialis Brevis (ECRB)). ECRL and ECRB tendons in the second dorsal compartment, Sax view of transducer placement and corresponding ultrasound images. ECRB (up arrow) and ECRL tendons (star), extensor retinaculum (down arrow), and Lister's tubercle (chevrons) are highlighted

- **Extensor Retinaculum, Third dorsal compartments (Extensor Pollicis Longus)**
  - Patient Position: seated with hand in pronation with palm resting on table.
  - Examiner Position: seated in front of the patient.
  - Probe Placement: Transverse plane over the radial side of the wrist.
  - Bony Acoustic Landmark(s): Lister's tubercle.
  - Target: The ECRB will be radial to Lister's tubercle while the EPL is ulnar to it. Once identified the EPL is followed on Sax plane to its insertion, highlighting its crossing over the ECRL and ECRB (Fig. 4.12).
- **Extensor Retinaculum, Fourth and Fifth dorsal compartments (Extensor Digitorum Communis, Extensor Indicis Proprius, and Extensor Digiti Minimi)**
  - Patient Position: seated with hand in pronation with palm resting on table.
  - Examiner Position: seated in front of the patient.
  - Probe Placement: Transverse plane over the middle of the wrist.

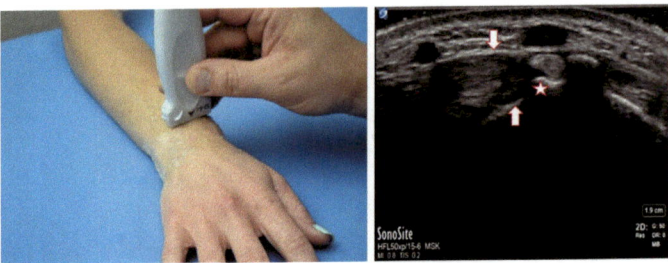

Fig. 4.12 Extensor retinaculum, Third dorsal compartments (Extensor Pollicis Longus). EPL tendon in the third dorsal compartment, Sax view of transducer placement and corresponding ultrasound images. EPL (up arrow), extensor retinaculum (down arrow), and Lister's tubercle (star) are highlighted

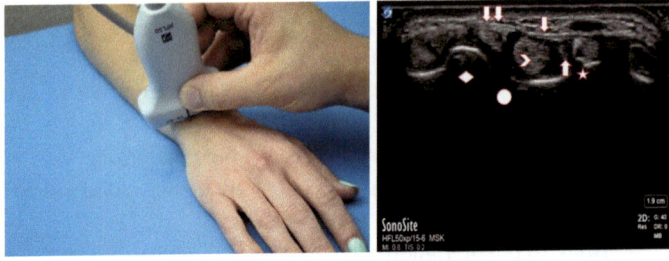

Fig. 4.13 Extensor retinaculum, fourth and fifth dorsal compartments (Extensor Digitorum Communis (EDC), Extensor Indicis Proprius (EIP), and Extensor Digiti Minimi (EDM)). EDC, EIP, and EDM tendons in the fourth and fifth dorsal compartments, Sax view of transducer placement and corresponding ultrasound images. EDC (chevron), EIP (up arrow), and EDM (below double down arrows) tendons, extensor retinaculum (down arrow), Lister's tubercle (star), ulna (diamond), and distal radioulnar joint (circle) are highlighted

- Bony Acoustic Landmark(s): Distal radius and ulna, radio-
  ulnar joint.
- Target: The EDC and EIP will be over the radius while the
  EDM will be over the ulna. The compartments and individual tendons in each of them can be identified easier with
  proper fingers flexion and extension. The EIP will be found
  deeper to the EDC in the fourth compartment (Fig. 4.13).

- **Distal posterior interosseous nerve (PIN)**
  - Patient Position: seated with hand pronated flat on the examination table.
  - Examiner Position: seated in front of the patient.
  - Probe Placement: dorsally on the distal interphalangeal joint of the assessed finger.
  - Probe Placement: Transverse plane over the middle of the wrist.
  - Bony Acoustic Landmark(s): Distal radius and ulna, radio-ulnar joint.
  - Target: The PIN is identified at the radial aspect of the fourth extensor compartment and appears as a noncompressible hypoechoic ovoid structure (Fig. 4.14).
- **Dorsal Scapholunate ligament**
  - Patient Position: seated with hand in pronation with palm resting on table, radial-ulnar deviation of the wrist facili-

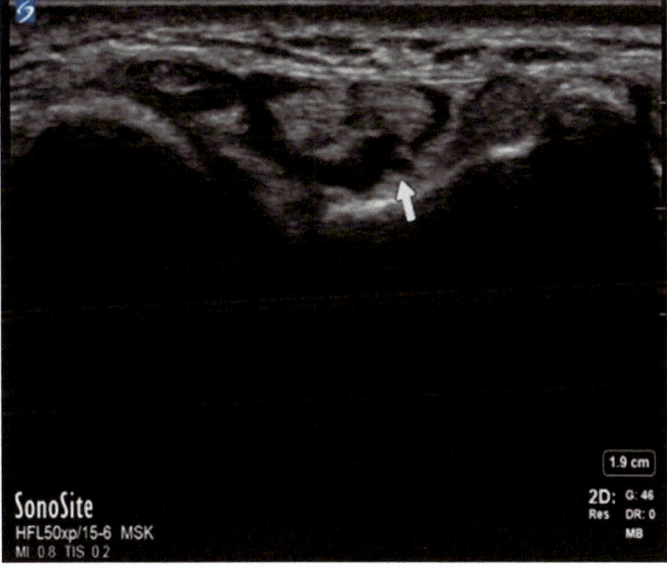

Fig. 4.14 Distal posterior interosseous nerve (PIN). PIN (arrow) can be seen at the radial aspect of the fourth extensor compartment

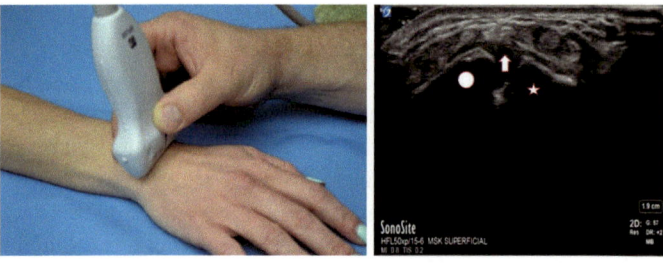

Fig. 4.15 Dorsal scapholunate ligament. Dorsal scapholunate ligament Lnx view of transducer placement and corresponding ultrasound images. Scapholunate ligament (arrow), scaphoid (star), and lunate (circle) are highlighted

tates assessment of the integrity of the ligament.
– Examiner Position: seated in front of the patient.
– Probe Placement: Transverse plane over Lister's tubercle.
– Bony Acoustic Landmark(s): Distal radius, Lister's tubercle, scaphoid, lunate.
– Target: Sweeping distally from Lister's tubercle, the dorsal component of the scapholunate ligament is identified; and in the hyperflexed hand—the proximal (or interosseous) component is visualized (Fig. 4.15).
• **Thumb UCL (Gamekeeper's Thumb assessment)**.
– Patient Position: seated, with hand grasping a rolled towel.
– Examiner Position: seated in front of the patient.
– Probe Placement: on the first metacarpophalangeal joint to obtain either a transverse or longitudinal image of the ulnar collateral ligament of the thumb (UCL).
– Bony Acoustic Landmark(s): first MCP joint.
– Target: The UCL of the thumb is assessed and can be found as a hyperechoic structure spanning the ulnar side of the first MCP joint. The normal UCL is subjacent to the adductor aponeurosis. Valgus stress tests can be applied to assess ligament's integrity (Fig. 4.16).
– Dynamic examination: Dynamic maneuvers such as clenching the fist or "curling" the thumb are helpful in assessing

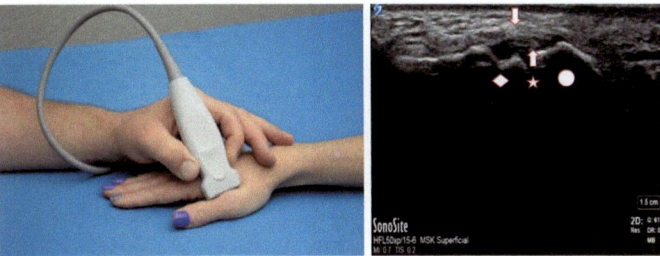

Fig. 4.16 Thumb Ulnar Collateral Ligament (UCL). UCL Lnx view of transducer placement and corresponding ultrasound images. UCL (up arrow), adductor aponeurosis (down arrow), first MCP joint (star), thumb metacarpal (diamond), and thumb proximal phalanx (circle) are highlighted

tendon stability and the location of the UCL underneath the adductor aponeurosis.

- **Extensor Hood/Sagittal band**
  - Patient Position: seated with hand pronated flat on the examination table and bolstered up by towel.
  - Examiner Position: seated in front of the patient.
  - Probe Placement: Sax dorsally on the metacarpophalangeal joint of the assessed finger.
  - Bony Acoustic Landmark(s): metacarpophalangeal joint of assessed finger.
  - Target: The sagittal band appears as a thin, echogenic structure that overlies the dorsal aspect of the MCP joint and extensor tendon. An irregular, thickening of the sagittal band with hypoechogenicity suggests ruptured sagittal band (Fig. 4.17).
  - Dynamic examination: The finger can be moved in extension and flexion, and the extensor tendon can be assessed for deviation to the ulnar or radial border of the MCP joint under extension in cases of sagittal band rupture. During full finger flexion, transverse sonogram will show dislocation of the extensor tendon on radial (usually) or ulnar side.

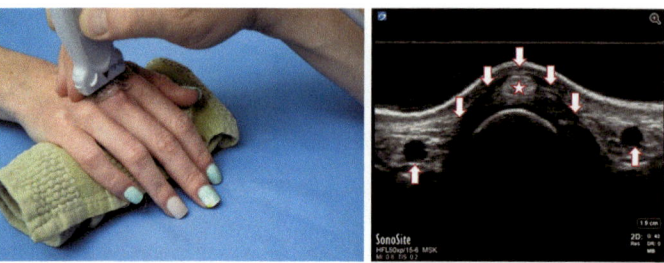

Fig. 4.17 Extensor hood/sagittal band. Extensor hood Sax view of transducer placement and corresponding ultrasound image. Extensor hood (down arrows), extensor digitorum tendon (star), and dorsal digital arteries (up arrows) are highlighted

- **Extensor Tendon at Finger level (Mallet Finger assessment)**
  - Patient Position: seated with hand pronated flat on the examination table.
  - Examiner Position: seated in front of the patient.
  - Probe Placement: dorsally on the distal interphalangeal joint of the assessed finger.
  - Bony Acoustic Landmark(s): distal interphalangeal joint of assessed finger.
  - Target: Begin at the base of the distal phalanx for assessment of extensor tendon integrity. The probe is moved proximally along the axis of the tendon and an irregular hypoechoic soft tissue lesion can be found over the distal shaft of the middle phalanx, indicative of the retracted tendon end. If an avulsion fracture is present, the detached bone fragment at the retracted tendon end and loss of substance in the distal phalangeal base can be detected.
- **Nail (Glomus apparatus/tumor assessment)**
  - Patient Position: seated with hand pronated flat on the examination table.
  - Examiner Position: seated in front of the patient.
  - Probe Placement: dorsally on the nail of interest.
  - Bony Acoustic Landmark(s): distal phalanx, and tuft.

- Target: Glomus tumor usually manifests as a nonspecific, solid, hypoechoic subungual mass. The underlying distal phalanx might contain sites of local erosion by the tumor. As the tumor is considered a hamartoma, hypervascularity at color Doppler imaging is expected.
- **Extensor Tendon Proximally (Boutonniere Deformity assessment)**
  - Patient Position: seated with hand pronated flat on the examination table.
  - Examiner Position: seated in front of the patient.
  - Probe Placement: dorsally on the middle interphalangeal joint of the assessed finger.
  - Bony Acoustic Landmark(s): middle interphalangeal joint of assessed finger.
  - Target: Begin at the base of the middle phalanx for assessment of extensor tendon integrity. The probe is moved proximally along the axis of the tendon and the central slip is identified. The lack of tendon echoes inserting into the middle phalangeal base and the presence of intact lateral slips on both sides of the middle phalanx are expected.

Notes
1. Lister's tubercle is a key bony landmark for the dorsal wrist evaluation.
2. All tendons can be traced proximally and distally as clinically indicated.

Ultrasound of the Hip

5

Anterior Region

- *Femoral head, neck, capsule, anterior synovial recess, and anterior labrum*
  - Patient Position: supine on table.
  - Examiner Position: seated on the side of the patient.
  - Probe Placement: in oblique Lnx over the femoral neck parallel to the femoral shaft (low frequency probe in obese patients).
  - Bony Acoustic Landmark(s): Femoral head.
  - Target: The femoral head is used as landmark to identify the anterior synovial recess. Proximal to the anterior recess, the acetabular anterior glenoid labrum can be detected as a homogeneously hyperechoic triangular fibrocartilaginous structure. The iliofemoral ligament can be identified superficial to the labrum (Fig. 5.1a, b).
- *Femoral vessels and nerve*
  - Patient Position: supine on table.
  - Examiner Position: seated on the side of the patient.
  - Probe Placement: in Sax over the inguinal region, perpendicular to femoral shaft.
  - Bony Acoustic Landmark(s): Joint space, femoral head.

© The Author(s), under exclusive license to Springer Nature Switzerland AG 2022
M. M. El-Othmani et al., *Sports Medicine and Musculoskeletal Ultrasound*, https://doi.org/10.1007/978-3-031-11764-0_5

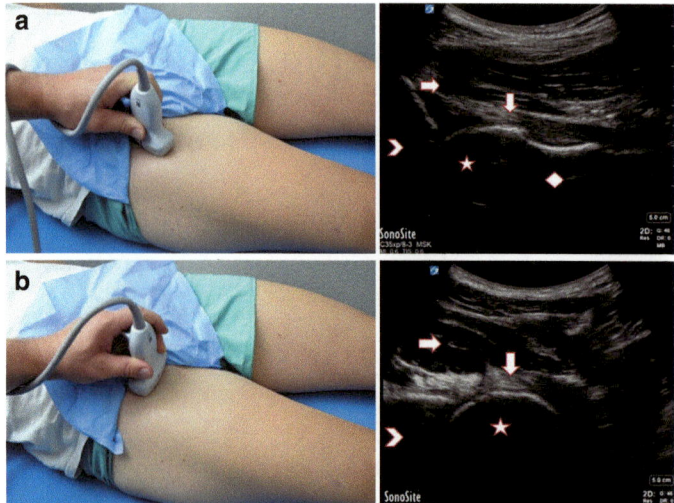

Fig. 5.1 Femoral head, neck, capsule, anterior synovial recess, anterior labrum, and iliopsoas muscle and tendon. Hip joint Sax view (**a**) and Lnx view (**b**) of transducer placement and corresponding ultrasound images. (**a**) and (**b**) Femoral head (star), neck (diamond), acetabulum (chevron), capsule (down arrows), and iliopsoas muscle complex (up arrows) are highlighted

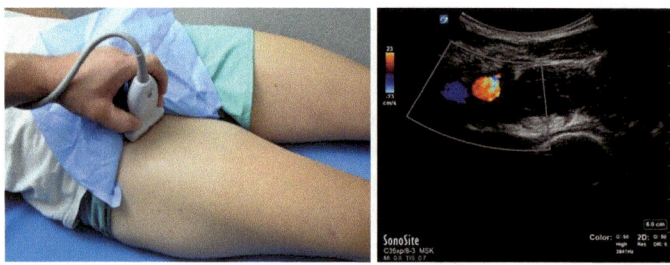

Fig. 5.2 Femoral vessels and nerve. Femoral neurovascular complex in Sax view with transducer placement and corresponding ultrasound images

- – Target: The femoral neurovascular bundle can be identified medial to the iliopsoas muscle and tendon. In the bundle, the femoral nerve will be lateral, while the common femoral artery and vein are medial (Fig. 5.2).

- – Dynamic Scanning: The vein and artery can be differentiated through the use of the Doppler function. Pressure application with probe would additionally compress the vein but not the artery.
- *Iliopsoas muscle, tendon, and bursa*
  - – Patient Position: supine on table.
  - – Examiner Position: seated on the side of the patient.
  - – Probe Placement: in Sax over the inguinal region, perpendicular to femoral shaft.
  - – Bony Acoustic Landmark(s): Joint space, femoral head.
  - – Target: The iliopsoas muscle is identified lateral to the femoral neurovascular bundle. At the iliopectineal eminence, the iliopsoas tendon is eccentric at the posterior and medial part of the muscle belly. The iliopsoas bursa lies between the tendon and the anterior capsule.
- *Sartorius and tensor fascia lata tendons and muscles*
  - – Patient Position: supine on table.
  - – Examiner Position: seated on the side of the patient.
  - – Probe Placement: in Sax over the anterior superior iliac spine (ASIS).
  - – Bony Acoustic Landmark(s): ASIS.
  - – Target: The sartorius tendon (medial) and the tensor fasciae latae (lateral) are identified as they originate from the ASIS (Fig. 5.3a, b).
  - – Scan-sweep: The probe is turned to the Lnx of the sartorius and followed medially to reach the medial thigh over the rectus femoris muscle. The same sweep can be performed over the tensor fasciae latae as it runs laterally and distally to insert into the anterior border of the fascia lata, superficial to the vastus lateralis.
- *Lateral femoral cutaneous nerve*
  - – Patient Position: supine on table.
  - – Examiner Position: seated on the side of the patient.
  - – Probe Placement: in Sax over the anterior superior iliac spine (ASIS).
  - – Bony Acoustic Landmark(s): ASIS.

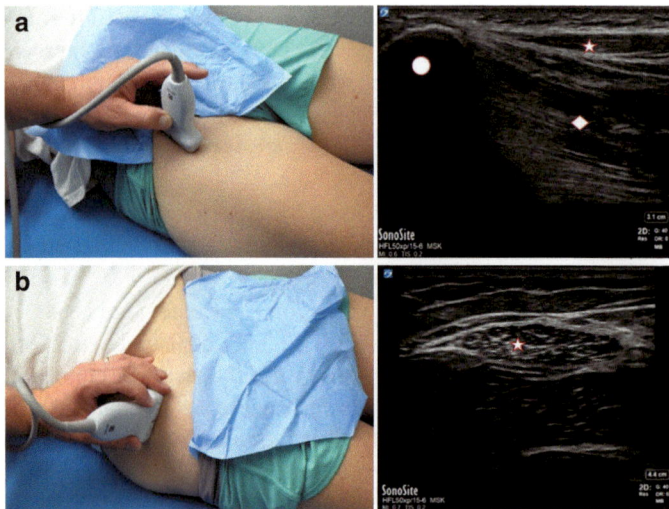

Fig. 5.3 Sartorius and tensor fascia lata tendons and muscles. Sartorius tendon and muscle Lnx view (**a**) and Sax view (**b**) of transducer placement and corresponding ultrasound images. (**a**) and (**b**) Sartorius (star), anterior superior iliac spine (circle), and iliopsoas muscle complex (diamond) are highlighted

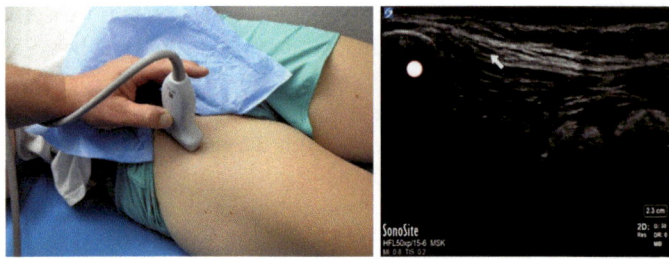

Fig. 5.4 Lateral femoral cutaneous nerve (LFCN). LFCN Lnx view of transducer placement and corresponding ultrasound images. LFCN (arrow) and anterior superior iliac spine (circle) are highlighted

  – Target: At the level of the ASIS, medial to the attachment of the inguinal ligament, the lateral femoral cutaneous nerve can be identified (Fig. 5.4).

- *Rectus femoris tendon(s) and muscles*
  - Patient Position: supine on table.
  - Examiner Position: seated on the side of the patient.
  - Probe Placement: in Sax over the anterior inferior iliac spine (AIIS).
  - Bony Acoustic Landmark(s): AIIS.
  - Target: The direct tendon of the rectus femoris can be identified as it originates from the AIIS (Fig. 5.5a, b).
  - Scan-sweep: The probe is turned to the Lnx of the direct tendon and followed distally. A posterior acoustic shadowing can be identified underlying the direct tendon. This shadowing is caused by the changes in tendon fibers orientation at the intersection of the direct and indirect tendons. Turning the probe to the Sax as the tendons is followed distally will locate the muscle belly as it enlarges between the tensor fasciae latae and the sartorius.

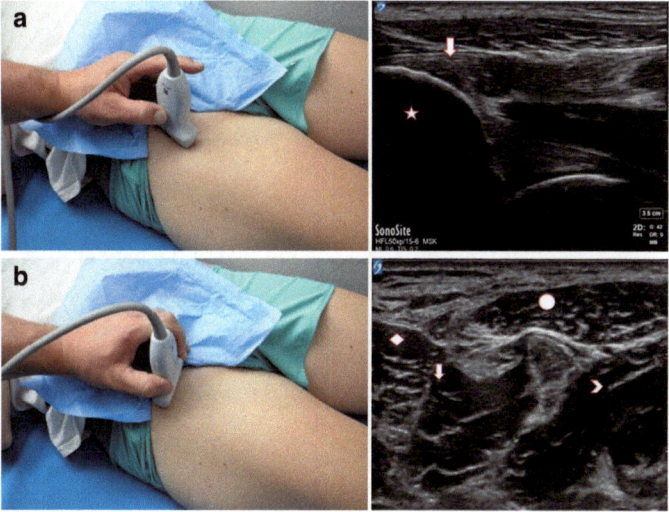

Fig. 5.5 Rectus femoris tendon and muscle. Rectus femoris tendon and muscle Lnx view (**a**) and Sax view (**a**) of transducer placement and corresponding ultrasound images. (**a**) and (**b**) Rectus femoris (down arrow), sartorius (circle), anterior superior iliac spine (star), tensor fascia latae (diamond), and iliopsoas muscle complex (chevron) are highlighted

Notes

1. Although several types of internal hip snapping may be detected during the anterior examination, most common is dyskinetic motion of the iliopsoas tendon at the level of the acetabular rim or hip joint. Symptoms are typically elicited while moving the hip from a flexed-abducted-externally rotated position to an extended-adducted-internally rotated position.

Lateral Region

- *Gluteus maximus and tensor fascia lata*
  - Patient Position: side lying on table with hip in 20–30 degrees of flexion.
  - Examiner Position: seated on the side of the patient.
  - Probe Placement: over the greater trochanter (GT).
  - Bony Acoustic Landmark(s): GT.
  - Target: The tensor fascia lata can be identified as a superficial hyperechoic band overlying the gluteus medius and minimus tendons at their insertion onto the GT. The gluteus maximus will be posterior to it (Fig. 5.6a, b).
- *Gluteus minimus tendon and muscle*
  - Patient Position: side lying on table with hip in 20–30 degrees of flexion.
  - Examiner Position: seated on the side of the patient.
  - Probe Placement: over the greater trochanter (GT).
  - Bony Acoustic Landmark(s): GT.
  - Target: The gluteus medius (superficial) and gluteus minimus (deep) muscle tendons can be identified as they insert at the GT (Fig. 5.6a, b).
  - Scan-sweep: The probe is shifted posteriorly from the tensor fasciae lata to identify the anterior margin of both muscles. Sweeping towards the GT the gluteus minimus tendon can be identified anteriorly as it inserts into the anterior facet of the GT.

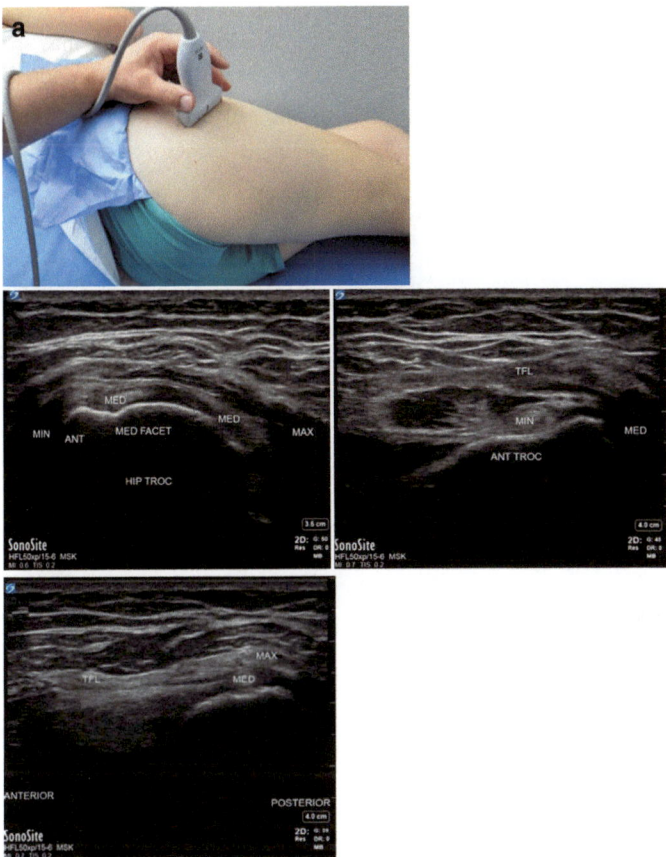

Fig. 5.6 Gluteus maximus, medius, minimus, and tensor fascia latae (TFL). Gluteus tendons and muscles and TFL Sax view (**a**) and Lnx view (**b**) of transducer placement and corresponding ultrasound images

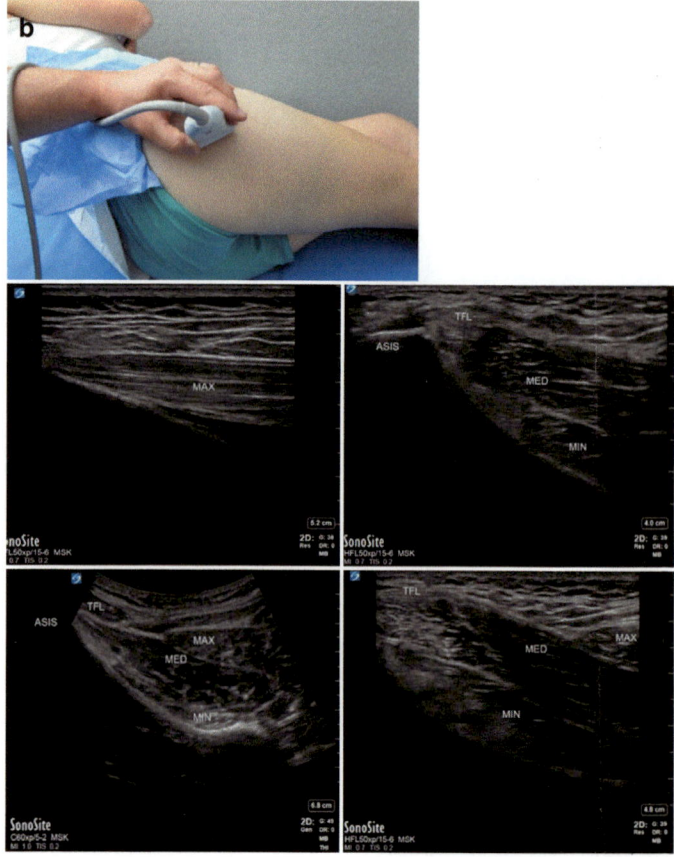

Fig. 5.6 (continued)

- *Gluteus medius tendon and muscle*
  - Patient Position: side lying on table with hip in 20–30 degrees of flexion.
  - Examiner Position: seated on the side of the patient.
  - Probe Placement: Lnx and Sax over the greater trochanter (GT).
  - Bony Acoustic Landmark(s): GT.

- Target: The gluteus medius (superficial) and gluteus minimus (deep) muscle tendons can be identified as they insert at the GT (Fig. 5.6a, b).
- Scan-sweep: The probe is placed over the lateral facet of the GT and the gluteus medius tendon can be identified as a curvilinear fibrillar band.
- *Greater trochanteric bursa (subgluteus maximus bursa)*
  - Patient Position: side lying on table with hip in 20–30 degrees of flexion.
  - Examiner Position: seated on the side of the patient.
  - Probe Placement: over the greater trochanter (GT), minimal pressure.
  - Bony Acoustic Landmark(s): GT.
  - Target: The bursae around the greater trochanter can be visualized in cases of inflammation and fluid collection (Fig. 5.7).
- *Dynamic scanning for snapping hip (as indicated)*

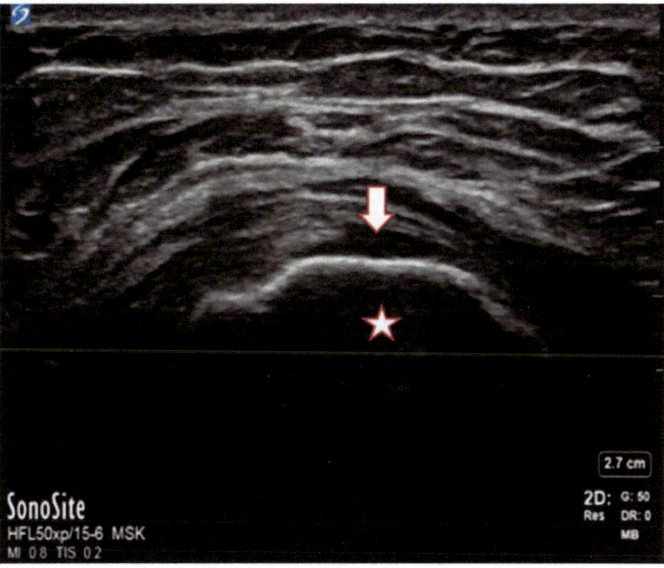

Fig. 5.7 Greater trochanteric bursa (subgluteus maximus bursa). Ultrasound image of the bursae (arrow) in Sax around the greater trochanter (star)

Notes
1. The most common cause of an external snapping hip is dyskinetic motion of the anterior gluteus maximus or iliotibial
   band, demonstrated during hip flexion-extension in a sidely-
   ing position.

Medial Region

- *Adductor muscles (Longus, gracilis, brevis, and magnus) and
  tendons*
  - Patient Position: supine on table with hips abducted and
    externally rotated while the knee is flexed (frog leg).
  - Examiner Position: seated on the side of the patient.
  - Probe Placement: Sax medially over the adductors.
  - Bony Acoustic Landmark(s): AIIS.
  - Target: The adductor longus (lateral) and the gracilis
    (medial) can be identified superficially, while the adductor
    brevis is located between the superficial group and the
    deeper adductor magnus (Fig. 5.8a, b).
  - Scan-sweep: The probe is turned into Lnx and the muscle
    are followed proximally to reach the origin at the pubis. The
    adductor longus insertion on the femur can be identified
    distally as a triangular hypoechoic shape.
- *Distal iliopsoas tendon*
  - Patient Position: supine on table with hips abducted and
    externally rotated while the knee is flexed (frog leg).
  - Examiner Position: seated on the side of the patient.
  - Probe Placement: in Lnx over the lesser trochanter.
  - Bony Acoustic Landmark(s): Lesser trochanter.
  - Target: The insertion of the iliopsoas tendon on the lesser
    trochanter can be assessed (Fig. 5.9).
- *Pubic bone, symphysis, and rectus abdominis muscle and
  tendon*
  - Patient Position: supine on table with hips abducted and
    externally rotated while the knee is flexed (frog leg).

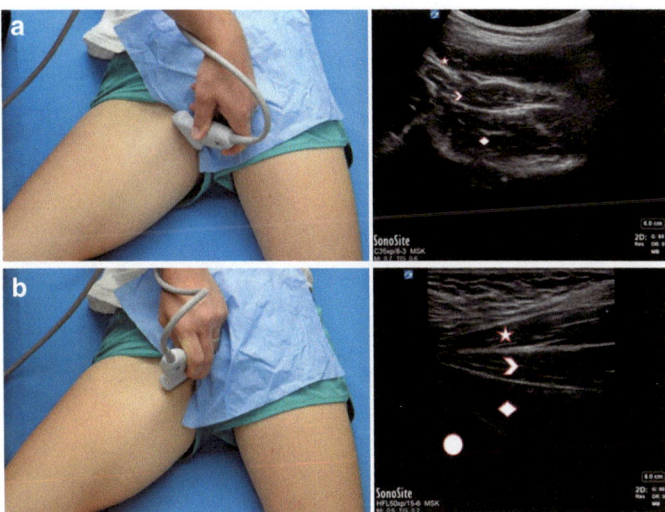

Fig. 5.8 Adductor muscles (longus, gracilis, brevis, and magnus) and tendons. Adductor muscles Sax view (**a**) and Lnx view (**b**) of transducer placement and corresponding ultrasound images. Pubic ramus (circle), adductor longus (star), brevis (chevron), and magnus (diamond) are highlighted

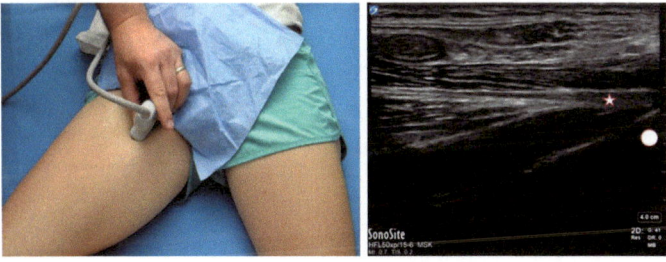

Fig. 5.9 Distal iliopsoas tendon. Iliopsoas at insertion Lnx view of transducer placement and corresponding ultrasound image. Lesser trochanter (circle) and iliopsoas tendon (star) are highlighted

- Examiner Position: seated on the side of the patient.
- Probe Placement: in oblique Lnx over the pubis.
- Bony Acoustic Landmark(s): Pubic symphysis.

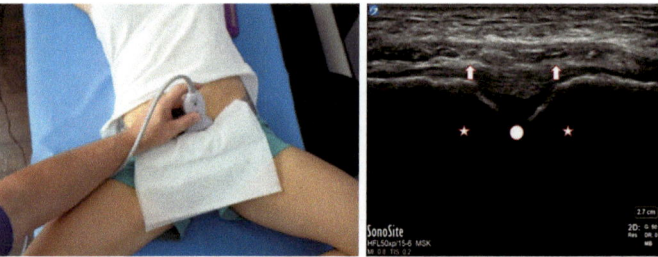

Fig. 5.10 Pubic bone, symphysis, and rectus abdominis muscle and tendon. Pubic symphysis Lnx view of transducer placement and corresponding ultrasound images. Conjoint tendon of transversus abdominis and internal oblique attachment (up arrows), symphysis pubis (stars), and joint space (circle) are highlighted

- – Target: The insertion of conjoint tendon of transversus abdominis and internal oblique can be assessed (Fig. 5.10).
- – Scan-sweep: The probe is moved medially until the anterior aspect of the symphysis pubis can be identified.

Notes
1. Initial identification of the adductor muscles in the short axis assists in their differentiation and facilitates the long-axis examination.
2. Evaluation for "athletic hernia" may involve additional examination in this region, including Valsalva and hernia evaluation.

Posterior Region

- • *Gluteus maximus muscle and tendon*
  - – Patient Position: lying prone on table with pillow under hips.
  - – Examiner Position: seated on the side of the patient.
  - – Probe Placement: just proximal to the gluteal fold (low frequency probe in obese patients).
  - – Bony Acoustic Landmark(s): ischial tuberosity.
  - – Target: The gluteus maximus muscle can be evaluated with Sax and Lnx views (Fig. 5.11).

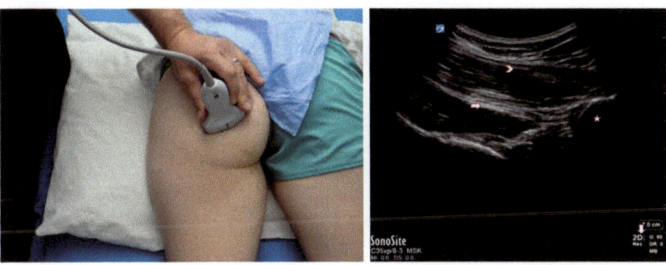

Fig. 5.11 Gluteus maximus and medius muscles and tendons. Gluteus tendons and muscles Lnx view of transducer placement and corresponding ultrasound images. Superoposterior aspect of greater trochanter (star), gluteus maximus (chevron), and gluteus medius tendon (arrow) are highlighted

- *Gluteus medius muscle and tendon*
  - Patient Position: lying prone on table with pillow under hips.
  - Examiner Position: seated on the side of the patient.
  - Probe Placement: just proximal to the gluteal fold (low frequency probe in obese patients).
  - Bony Acoustic Landmark(s): ischial tuberosity, GT.
  - Target: The posterior margin of the gluteus medius can be identified by moving the probe anteriorly from the anterior portion of the gluteus maximus. The tendon can be followed to its insertion at the GT (Fig. 5.11).
- *Deep short external rotators*
  - Patient Position: lying prone on table with pillow under hips.
  - Examiner Position: seated on the side of the patient.
  - Probe Placement: Sax low frequency probe just proximal to the gluteal fold.
  - Bony Acoustic Landmark(s): ischial tuberosity, sacroiliac joint.
  - Target: The sciatic nerve is identified as it emerges under the piriformis muscle. The piriformis can be followed to its insertion. The origin of the hamstring muscles on the lateral aspect of the ischial tuberosity is identified. The sciatic nerve can be assessed as a fascicular structure emerging under the piriformis muscle (Fig. 5.12).

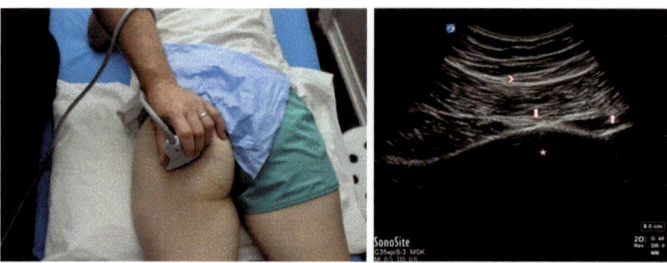

Fig. 5.12 Piriformis muscle and tendon. Deep short external rotators Lnx view of transducer placement and corresponding ultrasound images. Ilium (star), gluteus maximus (chevron), and piriformis muscle and tendon (up and down arrows, respectively) are highlighted

- – Scan-sweep: The short rotators can be assessed as the probe is moved distally after identifying the piriformis muscle.
- – Dynamic testing: The hip can be rotated internally and externally and the tendons motion is assessed.
- *Hamstring tendon and muscles (semimembranosus, semitendinosus, and biceps femoris)*
  - – Patient Position: lying prone on table with pillow under hips.
  - – Examiner Position: seated on the side of the patient.
  - – Probe Placement: just proximal to the gluteal fold.
  - – Bony Acoustic Landmark(s): ischial tuberosity.
  - – Target: The proximal origin of the ischiocrural (semimembranosus, semitendinosus, long head of the biceps femoris) muscles can be identified at the lateral aspect of the ischial tuberosity. The three tendons at this level cannot be separated (Fig. 5.13a, b).
  - – Scan-sweep: The hamstring tendons can be followed distally over the Sax. The tendon of semimembranosus can be identified superficial and lateral to the hyperechoic conjoined tendon of semitendinosus and biceps femoris. The muscle bellies of the semitendinosus (medial) and the biceps (lateral) are separated by the conjoined tendon.

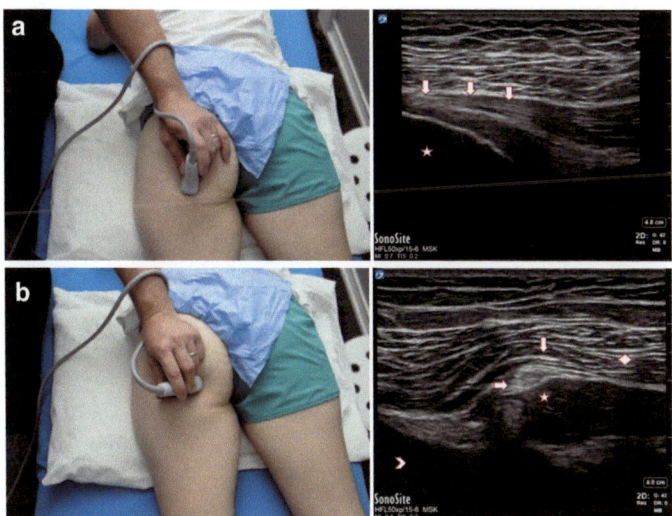

Fig. 5.13 Hamstring tendon and muscles (semimembranosus, semitendinosus, and biceps femoris). Hamstring muscles and tendons Lnx view (**a**) and Sax view (**b**) of transducer placement and corresponding ultrasound images. (**a**) Ischial tuberosity (star) and common tendon origin of the semitendinosus and long head of biceps femoris (down arrows). (**b**) Semitendinosus muscle (diamond) and tendon (down arrow), sciatic nerve (side arrow), adductor magnus (star), and femur (chevron) are highlighted

- *Ischial tuberosity and bursal region*
  - Patient Position: lying prone on table with pillow under hips.
  - Examiner Position: seated on the side of the patient.
  - Probe Placement: just proximal to the gluteal fold.
  - Bony Acoustic Landmark(s): ischial tuberosity.
  - Target: The ischial tuberosity is identified, and fluid collection superficial to the tuberosity in the bursal region can be identified in patients with bursitis (Fig. 5.13a).
- *Sciatic nerve*
  - Patient Position: lying prone on table with pillow under hips.

- Examiner Position: seated on the side of the patient.
- Probe Placement: just distal to the gluteal fold.
- Bony Acoustic Landmark(s): ischial tuberosity.
- Target: The origin of the hamstring muscles on the lateral aspect of the ischial tuberosity is identified. The sciatic nerve can be assessed as a fascicular structure emerging under the piriformis muscle.
- Scan-sweep: The nerve can be followed on the Lnx as it runs distally.

Notes

1. The gluteus minimus may not be visualized from the posterior view.
2. Examination of the deep short external rotators may include the piriformis, obturator internus-gemelli complex, and quadratus femoris.
3. Dynamic testing for ischiofemoral impingement can be performed as clinically indicated, with the transducer placed transversely along the long axis of the quadratus femoris during hip internal and external rotation.
4. The sciatic nerve emerges deep to the piriformis in most cases.
5. Evaluation of the sacroiliac joint can be performed as clinically indicated.

Ultrasound of the Knee

6

Anterior Knee Region

- *Quadriceps Tendon and Muscles.*
  - Patient Position: lying supine on table with pillow under knees to achieve 20–30 degrees of knee flexion.
  - Examiner Position: seated on the side of the patient.
  - Probe Placement: Lnx at midline just proximal to the patella.
  - Bony Acoustic Landmark(s): Patella.
  - Target: On Lnx the tendon has a multilayered typical hyperechoic fibrillary appearance. The tendon can be traced proximally over Sax to the myotendinous junction of the vastus lateralis, vastus medialis, deeper vastus intermedius, and more proximal rectus femoris (Fig. 6.1a and b).
  - Scan-sweep: The tendon should be assessed on Lnx and Sax while sweeping medially and laterally.
  - Dynamic testing: The knee is brought into flexion-extension to assess the integrity of all layers of the tendon.
- *Vastus Medialis and Medial Retinaculum (also with medial region scan).*
  - Patient Position: lying supine on table with pillow under knees to achieve 20–30 degrees of knee flexion, slight leg external rotation.

© The Author(s), under exclusive license to Springer Nature Switzerland AG 2022
M. M. El-Othmani et al., *Sports Medicine and Musculoskeletal Ultrasound*, https://doi.org/10.1007/978-3-031-11764-0_6

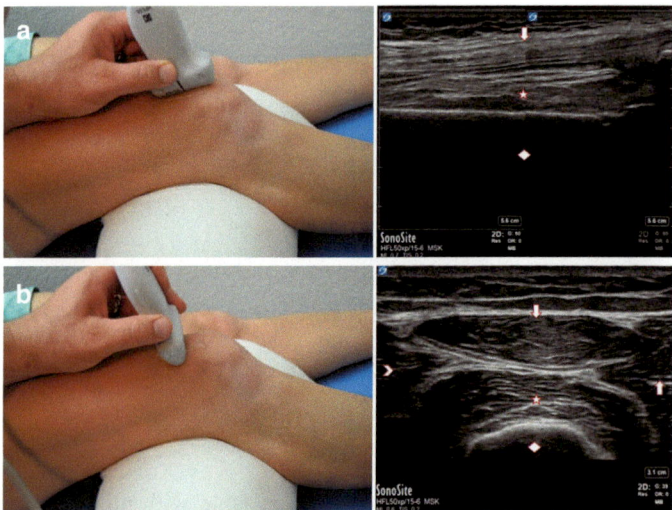

Fig. 6.1 Quadriceps Tendon and Muscles. Quadriceps muscles and tendons Lnx view (**a**) and Sax view (**b**) of transducer placement and corresponding ultrasound images. (**a**) The femur (diamond) and rectus femoris portion (arrow) and the vastus intermedius portion (star) of the quadriceps tendon are highlighted. Ischial tuberosity (star) and common tendon origin of the semitendinosus and long head of biceps femoris (down arrows) (**b**) The femur (diamond), rectus femoris (down arrow), vastus lateralis (up arrow), and vastus medialis (chevron) can be seen

- Examiner Position: seated on the side of the patient.
- Probe Placement: Lnx at midline just proximal to the patella.
- Bony Acoustic Landmark(s): Patella, femur.
- Target: The quadriceps tendon is identified and followed over Sax medially to identify vastus medialis myotendinous junction. The muscle can be followed proximally as needed. The medial retinaculum can be identified at its insertion on the medial patellar aspect as a bilayered structure and followed medially to posterior femoral aspect (Fig. 6.2).

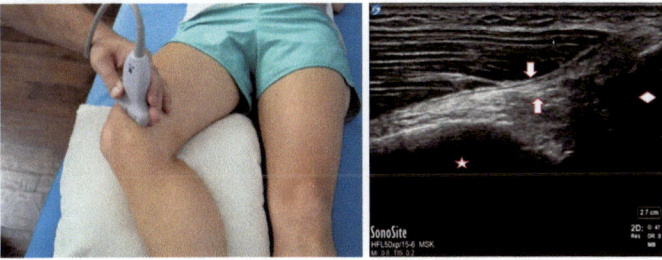

Fig. 6.2 Medial Retinaculum and patellofemoral ligament (also with medial regional scan). Sax view of transducer placement and corresponding ultrasound images. The femur (star), patella (diamond) and medial retinaculum (arrows) are highlighted

- *Vastus Lateralis and Lateral Retinaculum (also with lateral regional scan).*
  - Patient Position: lying supine on table with pillow under knees to achieve 20–30 degrees of knee flexion, slight leg internal rotation.
  - Examiner Position: seated on the side of the patient.
  - Probe Placement: Sax at midline just proximal to the patella.
  - Bony Acoustic Landmark(s): Patella, femur.
  - Target: The quadriceps tendon is identified and followed laterally to identify vastus lateralis myotendinous junction. The muscle can be followed proximally as needed. The lateral retinaculum can be identified at its insertion on the lateral patellar aspect as a bilayered structure and followed laterally (Fig. 6.3).
- *Suprapatellar recess of knee joint.*
  - Patient Position: lying supine on table with pillow under knees to achieve 20–30 degrees of knee flexion.
  - Examiner Position: seated on the side of the patient.
  - Probe Placement: Lnx at midline just proximal to the patella, minimal force applied.
  - Bony Acoustic Landmark(s): Patella.

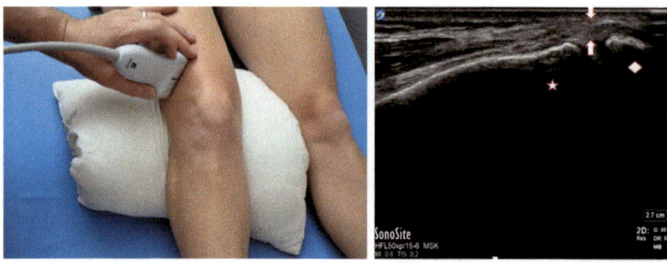

Fig. 6.3 Vastus Lateralis and Lateral Retinaculum (also with lateral regional scan). Sax view of transducer placement and corresponding ultrasound images. The femur (star), patella (diamond) and lateral retinaculum (arrows) are highlighted

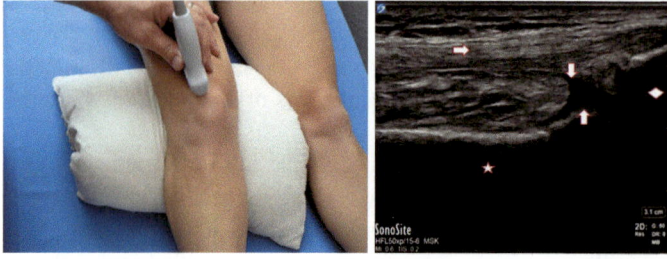

Fig. 6.4 Suprapatellar recess of knee joint. Lnx view of transducer placement and corresponding ultrasound images. The femur (star), patella (diamond), suprapatellar recess (arrows), and quadriceps tendon (horizontal arrow) are highlighted

- Target: The suprapatellar recess is identified deep to the distal third of the quadriceps tendon, just proximal to the patella, between the prefemoral and suprapatellar fat pads (appear as large hyperechoic spaces) (Fig. 6.4).
- Scan-sweep: Probe is moved over the quadriceps tendon laterally and medially.
- Dynamic testing: The knee is brought into additional flexion to drive any fluid into the recess.

- *Patella and Prepatellar Bursa.*
  - Patient Position: lying supine on table with pillow under knees to achieve 20–30 degrees of knee flexion.
  - Examiner Position: seated on the side of the patient.
  - Probe Placement: Lnx at midline over the patella, minimal pressure applied.
  - Bony Acoustic Landmark(s): Patella.
  - Target: The patella is identified and assessed, followed by assessment of the prepatellar bursa over the lower pole of the patella. The bursa should only be visible in cases of fluid collection (Fig. 6.5).
  - Scan-sweep: Probe is moved over the patella laterally and medially, from proximal to distal pole.
- *Patellar Tendon and Tibial Tubercle.*
  - Patient Position: lying supine on table with pillow under knees to achieve 20–30 degrees of knee flexion.
  - Examiner Position: seated on the side of the patient.
  - Probe Placement: Sax at midline at distal pole of the patella.
  - Bony Acoustic Landmark(s): Patella, proximal tibia.
  - Target: The tendon is identified at its origin at the inferior patellar pole as an echogenic fibrillar structure and followed distally to its insertion on the tibial tubercle (Fig. 6.6a and b).

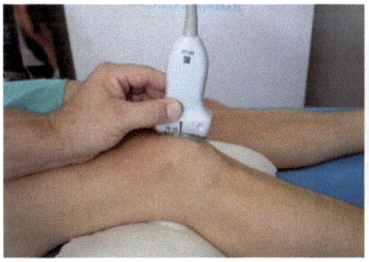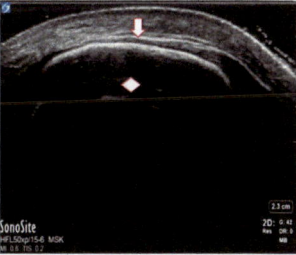

Fig. 6.5 Patella and Prepatellar Bursa. Patella and prepatellar bursa Lnx view of transducer placement and corresponding ultrasound images. The patella (diamond) and prepatellar bursa (arrow) are highlighted

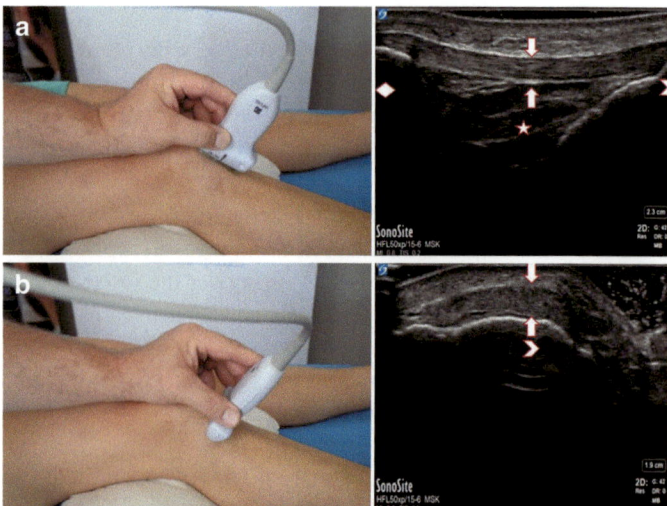

Fig. 6.6 Patellar Tendon and Tibial Tubercle. Patellar tendon Lnx view (**a**) and Sax view (**b**) of transducer placement and corresponding ultrasound images. (**a**) The patella (diamond), patellar tendon (arrows), Hoffa's fat pad (star), and tibial tubercle (chevron) are highlighted (**b**) The patellar tendon (arrows) and tibial tubercle (chevron) can be seen

- – Scan-sweep: Probe is moved over the patellar tendon later-
     ally and medially, from inferior pole of patella to tibial
     tubercle.
- – Dynamic testing: The knee is brought into flexion-extension
     to assess the integrity of the tendon.
- • *Superficial and Deep Infrapatellar Bursa.*
  - – Patient Position: lying supine on table with pillow under
       knees to achieve 20–30 degrees of knee flexion.
  - – Examiner Position: seated on the side of the patient.
  - – Probe Placement: Sax at midline inferior pole of patella,
       minimal force applied.
  - – Bony Acoustic Landmark(s): Patella.
  - – Target: Deep infrapatellar bursa can be identified deep to
       the patellar tendon and superficial to the tibia as a triangular
       hypoechoic area. The superficial infrapatellar bursa should
       not be visible in normal subjects.

- *Distal Femoral Cartilage (as indicated).*
  - Patient Position: lying supine on table with knee in 90 degrees of flexion.
  - Examiner Position: seated on the side of the patient.
  - Probe Placement: Sax at midline just proximal to the patella.
  - Bony Acoustic Landmark(s): Patella, femoral trochlea.
  - Target: Femoral trochlear cartilage appears as a hypoechoic structure with uniform thickness (Fig. 6.7a, b, and c).
  - Scan-sweep: Probe is moved laterally and medially.

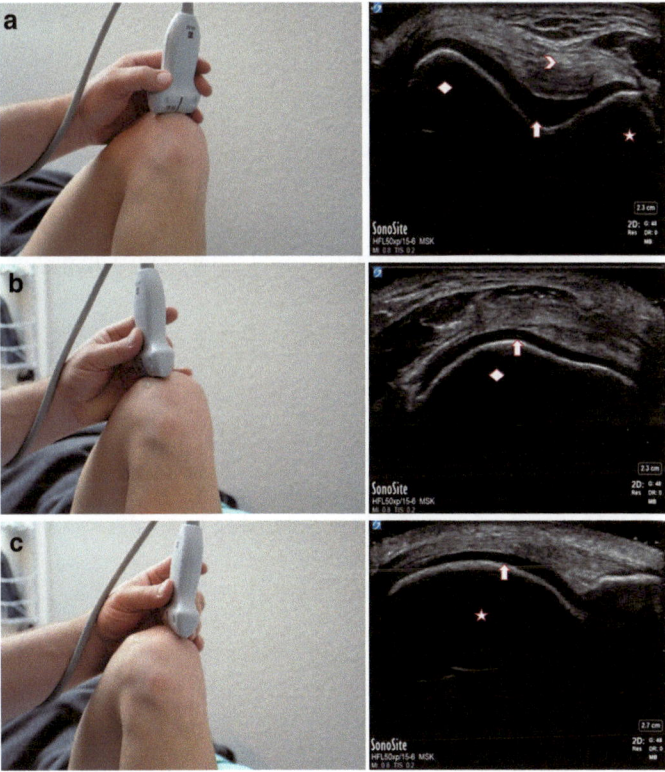

Fig. 6.7 Distal Femoral Cartilage. Distal femoral cartilage Sax view (**a**) and Lnx view (lateral (**b**) and medial (**c**) condyles) of transducer placement and corresponding ultrasound images. The lateral condyle (diamond), medial condyle (star), cartilage (arrow), and quadriceps tendon (chevron) are highlighted

Notes

1. Examination for superficial bursa may require a standoff pad or heaping gel on the skin to minimize transducer pressure and the possibility of a false negative examination.
2. Dynamic examination for the quadriceps and patellar tendons may include transducer pressure, passive or active knee flexion, active quadriceps contraction, patellar glides, or resisted knee extension. The maneuvers may assist in the identification of partial or full thickness tears.

Medial Knee Region

- *Medial Collateral Ligament.*
    - Patient Position: lying supine on table with leg externally rotated and knee flexed to 20–30 degrees, with pillow under lateral side.
    - Examiner Position: seated on the side of the patient.
    - Probe Placement: Lnx at the distal femur with a 45 degrees tilt to the shaft of the femur.
    - Bony Acoustic Landmark(s): medial femoral condyle, proximal tibia.
    - Target: On Lnx the MCL can be identified as a bulky hypoechoic fibrillar tissue (Fig. 6.8a and b).
    - Scan-sweep: The ligament should be assessed on Lnx and Sax while sweeping medially and laterally.
    - Dynamic testing: The knee is brought into valgus to assess the integrity of the ligament.
- *Medial Meniscus and Medial Tibiofemoral Joint Space.*
    - Patient Position: lying supine on table with leg externally rotated and knee flexed to 20–30 degrees, with pillow under lateral side.
    - Examiner Position: seated on the side of the patient.
    - Probe Placement: Lnx at the medial joint line.
    - Bony Acoustic Landmark(s): medial femoral condyle, proximal tibia.

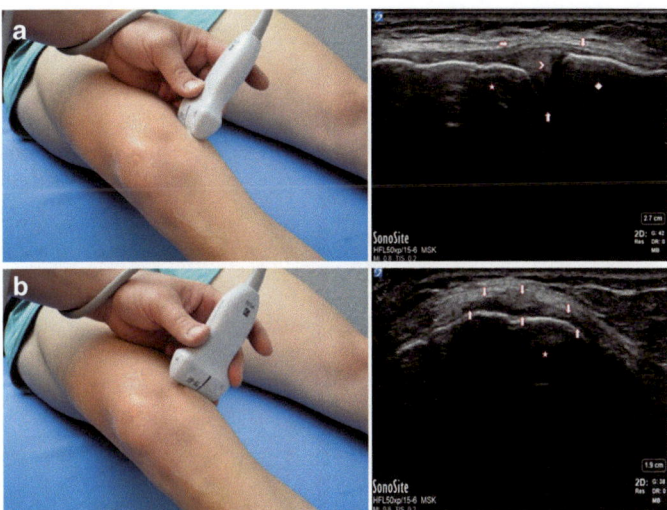

Fig. 6.8 Medial Collateral Ligament (MCL), Medial Meniscus and Medial Tibiofemoral Joint Space. MCL Lnx view (**a**) and Sax view (**b**) of transducer placement and corresponding ultrasound images. (**a**) The tibia (diamond), femur (star), superficial (horizontal arrow) and deep (down arrow) MCL, medial tibiofemoral joint space (up arrow) and meniscus (chevron) are highlighted. (**b**) The femur (star) and MCL (arrows) can be seen

- – Target: The medial meniscus and tibiofemoral joint space can be identified just deep to the MCL. The medial meniscus will appear as a triangular and hyperechoic structure.
- – Scan-sweep: The probe can be moved slightly anteriorly to visualize the anterior horn of the medial meniscus.
- *Pes Anserine Tendons and Bursa.*
  - – Patient Position: lying supine on table with leg externally rotated and knee flexed to 20–30 degrees, with pillow under lateral side.
  - – Examiner Position: seated on the side of the patient.
  - – Probe Placement: Sax at the distal femur, minimal pressure applied.
  - – Bony Acoustic Landmark(s): distal femur, proximal tibia.

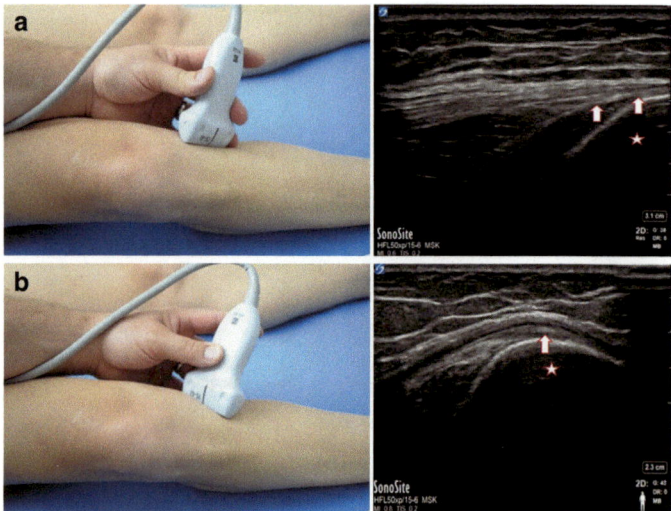

Fig. 6.9 Pes Anserine Tendons and Bursa. Pes anserine Lnx view (**a**) and Sax view (**b**) of transducer placement and corresponding ultrasound images. The tibia (star) and pes anserine tendon complex (up arrows) are highlighted

- – Target: On Sax the MCL is identified and the tendons of sartorius (most anterior), gracilis, and semitendinosus (most posterior) are identified and followed to the insertion at the pes anserine. At the pes, the bursa can be assessed for any fluid collection (Fig. 6.9a and b).
- – Scan-sweep: The tendons should be assessed on Lnx and Sax while sweeping proximally to distally.
- • *Medial Patellar Retinaculum and Patellofemoral Joint (also with anterior region scan).*
  - – Patient Position: lying supine on table with leg externally rotated and knee extended.
  - – Examiner Position: seated on the side of the patient.
  - – Probe Placement: Lnx at the medial superior aspect of the patella.
  - – Bony Acoustic Landmark(s): medial femoral condyle, medial patella.

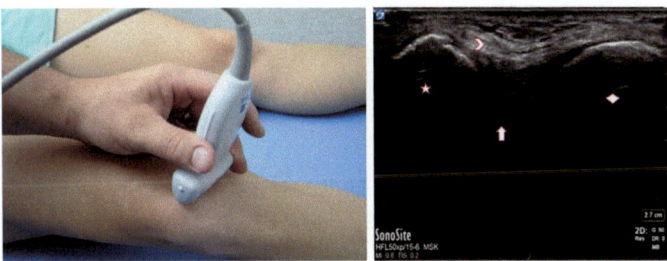

Fig. 6.10 Medial Patellar Retinaculum and Patellofemoral Joint. Medial Patellar Retinaculum Sax view of transducer placement and corresponding ultrasound images. The medial condyle (diamond), patella (star), medial patellofemoral joint (up arrow) and medial retinaculum (chevron) can be seen

- Target: On Lnx the medial patellar retinaculum at its insertion on the upper third of the medial patella, and can be followed to its origin from the posterior aspect of the medial femoral condyle. The patellofemoral joint space can be identified deeper (Fig. 6.10).
- Scan-sweep: The retinaculum should be assessed on Lnx and Sax while sweeping over its course.
- Dynamic testing: Lateral tilt of the patella can be applied to assess the integrity of the retinaculum.

Notes
1. The pes tendons may be identified at the posterior-posteromedial knee and traced distally to the pes.
2. Valgus stress testing is typically performed at 30 degrees of knee flexion.

Lateral Knee Region

- *Iliotibial Band.*
  - Patient Position: lying supine on table with leg internally rotated and knee flexed to 20–30 degrees, with pillow supporting medial side.
  - Examiner Position: seated on the side of the patient.

- Probe Placement: Lnx at the distal femur parallel to the shaft of the femur/axis of the thigh.
- Bony Acoustic Landmark(s): lateral femoral condyle, proximal tibia.
- Target: On Lnx the IT band can be identified as a thin flat hypoechoic fibrillar structure (Fig. 6.11).
- Scan-sweep: The IT band should be assessed on Lnx and Sax while sweeping medially and laterally, and followed to its insertion on Gerdy tubercle at the tibia.

• *Lateral Collateral Ligament.*
  - Patient Position: lying supine on table with leg internally rotated and knee flexed to 20–30 degrees, with pillow supporting medial side.
  - Examiner Position: seated on the side of the patient.
  - Probe Placement: Lnx at the distal femur parallel to the shaft of the femur/axis of the thigh.
  - Bony Acoustic Landmark(s): lateral femoral condyle, fibular head.
  - Target: The LCL can be identified as hypoechoic fibrillar structure extending from the lateral femoral condyle to the head of the fibula (Fig. 6.12).
  - Scan-sweep: The ligament should be assessed on Lnx and Sax while sweeping proximally and distally.

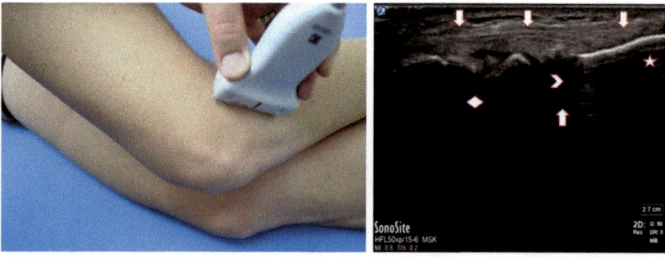

Fig. 6.11 Iliotibial Band (IT Band), Lateral Meniscus, and Lateral Tibio-femoral Joint Space. Lateral tibiofemoral joint space and IT band in Lnx view of transducer placement and corresponding ultrasound images. The tibial gerdy's tubercle (star), femur (diamond), lateral meniscus (chevron), lateral tibiofemoral joint space (up arrow), and IT band (down arrow) are highlighted

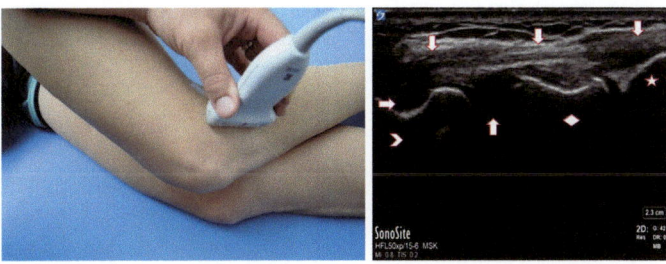

Fig. 6.12 Lateral Collateral Ligament (LCL) and Popliteus tendon. LCL in Lnx view of transducer placement and corresponding ultrasound images. The fibula (star), tibia (diamond), femur (chevron), lateral tibiofemoral joint space (up arrow), popliteus tendon (horizontal arrow), and LCL (down arrow) are highlighted

- Dynamic testing: The knee is brought into varus stress to assess the integrity of the ligament.
- *Lateral Meniscus and Tibiofemoral Joint Space.*
  - Patient Position: lying supine on table with leg internally rotated and knee flexed to 20–30 degrees, with pillow supporting medial side.
  - Examiner Position: seated on the side of the patient.
  - Probe Placement: Lnx at the lateral tibiofemoral joint line.
  - Bony Acoustic Landmark(s): lateral femoral condyle, proximal tibia.
  - Target: The lateral meniscus and tibiofemoral joint space can be identified deep to the IT band. The lateral meniscus will appear as a triangular and hyperechoic structure.
  - Scan-sweep: The probe can be moved slightly anteriorly to visualize the anterior horn of the lateral meniscus.
- *Biceps Femoris Tendon and Muscles.*
  - Patient Position: lying supine on table with leg internally rotated and knee flexed to 20–30 degrees, with pillow supporting medial side.
  - Examiner Position: seated on the side of the patient.
  - Probe Placement: Lnx at the distal femur parallel with distal end of the probe over the head of the fibula.
  - Bony Acoustic Landmark(s): lateral femoral condyle, fibular head.

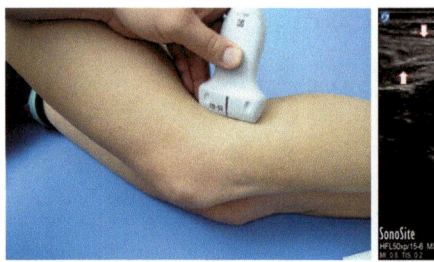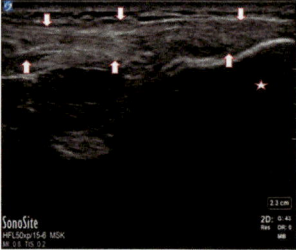

Fig. 6.13 Biceps Femoris Tendon and Muscles. Biceps femoris tendon Lnx view of transducer placement and corresponding ultrasound images. The fibula (star) and biceps femoris (arrows) are highlighted

- Target: The biceps femoris tendon can be identified as it courses posteriorly in relation to the LCL and inserts at the head of the fibula (Fig. 6.13).
- Scan-sweep: The tendon should be assessed on Lnx and Sax while sweeping proximally and distally.
- *Popliteus Tendon and muscle.*
    - Patient Position: lying supine on table with leg internally rotated and knee flexed to 20–30 degrees, with pillow supporting medial side.
    - Examiner Position: seated on the side of the patient.
    - Probe Placement: Lnx at the distal femur parallel to the shaft of the femur/axis of the thigh.
    - Bony Acoustic Landmark(s): lateral femoral condyle, proximal tibia.
    - Target: Identify the IT band and move the probe laterally until the groove for the popliteal tendon in the lateral femoral condyle is visualized, deep to the LCL (Fig. 6.12).
    - Scan-sweep: The tendon can be followed as it turns posteriorly around the joint, and can be followed distally to identify the muscle belly over the posterior aspect of the tibia.
    - Dynamic testing: The knee can be rotated internally and externally and the tendons motion is assessed.
- *Lateral Patellar Retinaculum and Patellofemoral Joint.*
    - Patient Position: lying supine on table with leg internally rotated and knee extended.

- Examiner Position: seated on the side of the patient.
- Probe Placement: Lnx at the lateral superior aspect of the patella.
- Bony Acoustic Landmark(s): lateral femoral condyle, lateral patella.
- Target: On Lnx the lateral patellar retinaculum at its insertion on the lateral patella, and can be followed to its origin at the femoral condyle. The lateral patellofemoral joint space can be identified deeper.
- Scan-sweep: The retinaculum should be assessed on Lnx and Sax while sweeping over its course.
- *Proximal Tibiofibular Joint.*
  - Patient Position: lying supine on table with leg internally rotated and knee extended.
  - Examiner Position: seated on the side of the patient.
  - Probe Placement: at the head of the fibula and directed towards the inferior pole of the patella.
  - Bony Acoustic Landmark(s): lateral tibial plateau, fibular head.
  - Target: A thick anterior superior tibiofibular ligament should be identified, and the joint space will be just deep to it (Fig. 6.14).

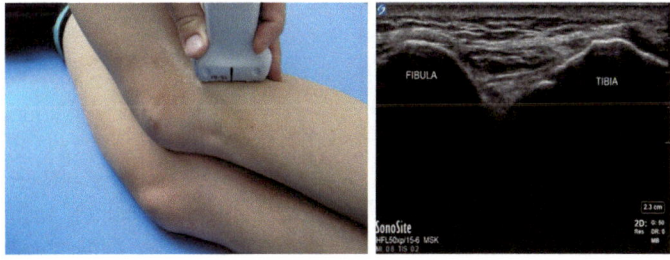

Fig. 6.14 Proximal Tibiofibular Joint. Tibiofibular joint Lnx view of transducer placement and corresponding ultrasound images

Notes

1. Varus stress testing is typically performed at 30 degrees of knee flexion.
2. Iliotibial band motion may be dynamically assessed during flexion-extension at the level of the lateral femoral epicondyle while visualizing the ITB in its short axis.

Posterior Knee Region

- *Popliteal Fossa, Artery, and Vein.*
  - Patient Position: lying prone on table with knee extended.
  - Examiner Position: seated on the side of the patient.
  - Probe Placement: in Sax over the popliteal fold, minimal pressure applied.
  - Bony Acoustic Landmark(s): posterior femur, posterior tibia.
  - Target: In the fossa, the popliteal artery can be found deep to the more superficial popliteal vein (Fig. 6.15a and b).
  - Scan-sweep: Sweep the probe proximal to distal over the popliteal neurovascular bundle.
  - Dynamic testing: If the vein can't be identified, slight flexion of the knee is performed allowing the vein to fill and improve its detection. Doppler function can be used to facilitate differentiation of the vein and artery (Fig. 6.15a and b).
- *Sciatic, Tibial, and Common Fibular Nerves.*
  - Patient Position: lying prone on table with knee extended.
  - Examiner Position: seated on the side of the patient.
  - Probe Placement: high-frequency linear-array probe in Sax over the popliteal fold.
  - Bony Acoustic Landmark(s): Posterior femur, posterior tibia.
  - Target: The sciatic nerve can be identified proximal to the apex of the popliteal space and followed distally. At the space, the nerve will bifurcate to provide the tibial nerve medially and common fibular nerve laterally. The tibial nerve can be identified superficial to the popliteal artery and

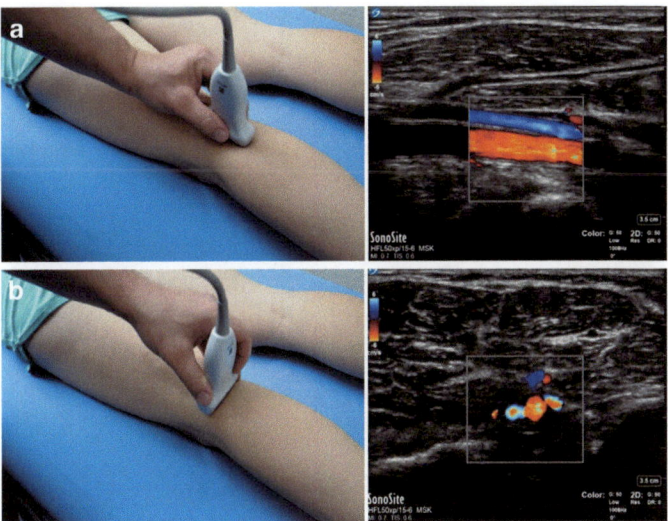

Fig. 6.15 Popliteal Fossa, Artery, and Vein. Popliteal artery and vein Lnx view (**a**) and Sax view (**b**) of transducer placement and corresponding ultrasound images with Doppler function deployed

vein. In Lnx, the nerves can be seen as coarse and hypoechoic structures, and have a honeycomb appearance in Sax (Fig. 6.16a).

- Scan-sweep: Sweep the probe proximal to distal over the popliteal neurovascular bundle on Lnx (Fig. 6.16a) and Sax (Fig. 6.16b). The common fibular nerve can be followed as it turns around the neck of the fibula.

• *Medial Head of Gastrocnemius Tendon and Muscle, Semimembranosus Tendon and Muscle, Semimembranosus-Gastrocnemius Bursa, and Semitendinosus Tendon.*

- Patient Position: lying prone on table with knee extended.
- Examiner Position: seated on the side of the patient.
- Probe Placement: in Sax over the medial aspect of the mid-calf region, light pressure applied.
- Bony Acoustic Landmark(s): Posterior femoral condyle.
- Target: The medial head of gastrocnemius muscle is identified in the mid-calf as it lies superficial to the soleus muscle.

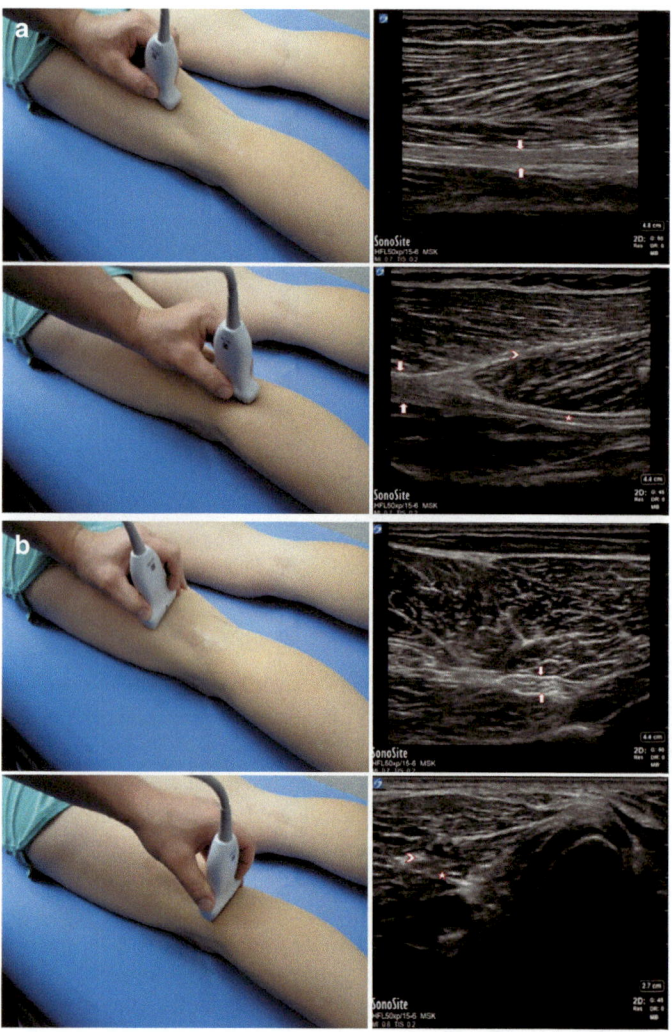

Fig. 6.16 Sciatic, Tibial, and Common Fibular Nerves. Posterior nerves in Lnx view (**a**) and Sax view (**b**) of transducer placement and corresponding ultrasound images. The sciatic nerve (between arrows), tibial nerve (star), and common peroneal nerve (chevron) are highlighted

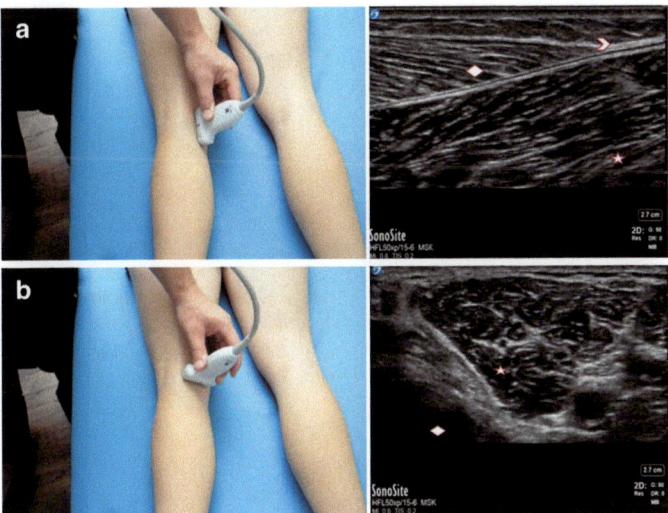

Fig. 6.17 Medial Head of Gastrocnemius Tendon and Muscle, Semimembranosus Tendon and Muscle, Semimembranosus-Gastrocnemius Bursa, and Semitendinosus Tendon. Medial head of gastrocnemius Lnx view (**a**) and Sax view (**b**) of transducer placement and corresponding ultrasound images. (**a**) The medial gastrocnemius (star), semimembranosus (diamond), and semitendinosus (chevron) are highlighted. (**b**) The femoral condyle (diamond) and medial gastrocnemius (star) can be seen

The muscle can then be traced proximally to the level of the popliteal fossa, until the posterior femoral condyle is visualized. At this level, the semimembranosus tendon can be identified as it lies just medial to the gastrocnemius, and separated from it by the bursal space. The semitendinosus tendon is identified superficial to the semimembranosus tendon (Fig. 6.17a and b).

- – Scan-sweep: Sweep the probe proximal to distal in Lnx and Sax to trace the tendons and muscles as needed.
- • *Lateral Gastrocnemius Muscle and Tendon.*
  - – Patient Position: lying prone on table with knee extended.
  - – Examiner Position: seated on the side of the patient.

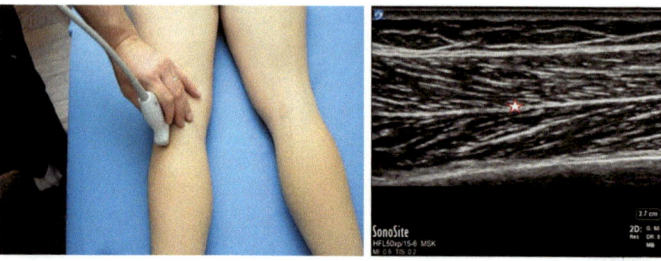

Fig. 6.18 Lateral Gastrocnemius Muscle and Tendon. Lateral head of gastrocnemius Lnx view of transducer placement and corresponding ultrasound images. The medial gastrocnemius (star), semimembranosus (diamond), and semitendinosus (chevron) are highlighted

- Probe Placement: in Sax over the lateral aspect of the mid-calf region.
- Bony Acoustic Landmark(s): posterior femoral condyle.
- Target: The lateral head of gastrocnemius muscle is identified in the mid-calf as it lies superficial to the soleus muscle. The muscle can then be traced proximally to the level of the popliteal fossa, until the posterior femoral condyle is visualized (Fig. 6.18).
- Scan-sweep: Sweep the probe proximal to distal in Lnx and Sax to trace the tendon and muscle as needed.
- *Posterior Horns of Medial and Lateral Menisci and Tibiofemoral Joint Space.*
  - Patient Position: lying prone on table with knee extended.
  - Examiner Position: seated on the side of the patient.
  - Probe Placement: low frequency in Sax over the medial and lateral popliteal fold.
  - Bony Acoustic Landmark(s): Posterior femur, posterior tibia.
  - Target: The posterior horn of the medial and lateral menisci can be identified on the medial and lateral sides, respectively. The menisci will appear as triangular and hyperechoic structures.

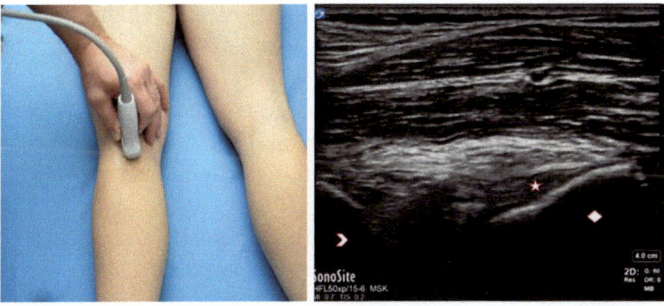

Fig. 6.19 Posterior Cruciate Ligament (PCL). PCL Lnx view of transducer placement and corresponding ultrasound images. The PCL (star), tibia (diamond), and femur (chevron) are highlighted

- Dynamic testing: The knee can be brought into flexion and the menisci can be assessed for excursion.
- *Posterior Cruciate Ligament.*
  - Patient Position: lying prone on table with knee extended.
  - Examiner Position: seated on the side of the patient.
  - Probe Placement: low frequency at 45 degrees over the midline popliteal fold, with distal portion of the probe towards the lateral tibial plateau.
  - Bony Acoustic Landmark(s): Posterior medial femur, posterior lateral tibia.
  - Target: The mid-distal portion of the PCL can be identified deep in the intercondylar fossa (Fig. 6.19).
  - Scan-sweep: Sweep the probe proximal to distal over the ligament to its insertion.
  - Dynamic testing: Applying posteriorly directed force over the tibia will stress the ligament and help in assessment of its integrity.

Notes

1. A Baker's cyst is a specific type of popliteal cyst which represents distention of the medial gastrocnemius-semimembranosus bursa. A Baker's cyst should be diagnosed only when a com-

municative stalk with the posterior tibiofemoral joint is visualized extending between the medial gastrocnemius and semimembranosus.

2. The tibial vein is often compressed and therefore not visualized secondary to transducer pressure. To see the vein, which occasionally may be duplicated, light transducer pressure is required.

3. The tibial nerve, vein, and artery are visualized superficial to deep in the posterior-posterolateral portion of the popliteal fossa.

Ultrasound of the Ankle and Foot

7

Anterior Ankle Region

1. *Tibialis anterior muscle and tendon.*
   a. Patient Position: lying supine on table with foot free at distal edge of the table.
   b. Examiner Position: seated in front of the patient.
   c. Probe Placement: Sax medial at the level of the ankle joint.
   d. Bony Acoustic Landmark(s): medial distal tibia, talus.
   e. Target: The tibialis anterior tendon is largest and most medial of the anterior region tendons, and can be seen as a fibrillary structure on Lnx and as a hyperechoic structure with speckled pattern appearance on Sax (Fig. 7.1a and b).
   f. Scan-sweep: The probe can be moved proximally and distally on Lnx and Sax to trace the tendon from the anterolateral musculotendinous junction as it follows an oblique inferomedial path to insert on anteromedial aspect of the medial cuneiform and base of first metatarsal.
   g. Dynamic testing: The ankle is brought into dorsiflexion and plantarflexion to assess the integrity of the tendon.
2. *Extensor Hallucis Longus (EHL) tendon and muscle.*
   a. Patient Position: lying supine on table with foot free at distal edge of the table.
   b. Examiner Position: seated in front of the patient.

© The Author(s), under exclusive license to Springer Nature Switzerland AG 2022
M. M. El-Othmani et al., *Sports Medicine and Musculoskeletal Ultrasound*, https://doi.org/10.1007/978-3-031-11764-0_7

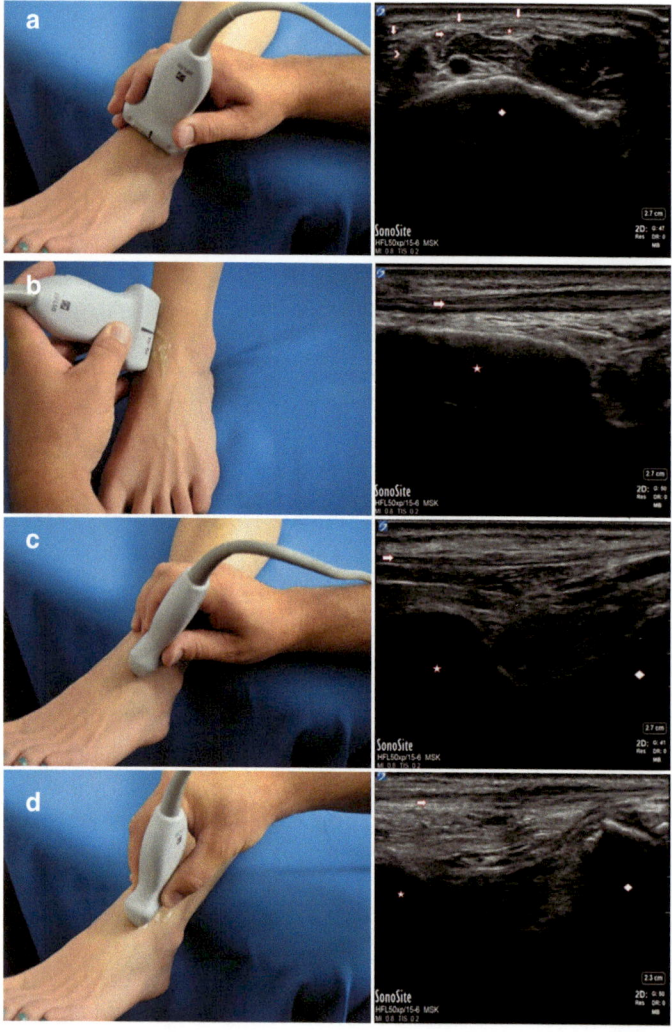

Fig. 7.1 Tibialis anterior (TA), Extensor Hallucis Longus (EHL), Extensor Digitorum Longus (EDL) muscles and tendons, and Superior Extensor Retinaculum. TA, EHL, and EDL muscles and tendons (Sax and Lnx). Sax view (**a**) and Lnx view (**b, c**), and (**d**) of transducer placement and corresponding ultrasound images. (**a**) TA (chevron), EHL (horizontal arrow), EDL (star), superior extensor retinaculum (down arrows), and talus (diamond) can be seen. (**b**) Tibia (star) and TA (horizontal arrow). (**c**) Tibia (star), Talus (diamond) and EHL (horizontal arrow). (**d**) Tibia (star), Talus (diamond) and EDL (horizontal arrow)

c. Probe Placement: Sax medial to midline at the level of the ankle joint.

d. Bony Acoustic Landmark(s): distal tibia, talus.

e. Target: Once the tibialis anterior tendon is identified, the EHL is just lateral to it and can be identified as a smaller tendon with a fibrillary appearance on Lnx and as a hyperechoic structure with speckled pattern appearance on Sax (Fig. 7.1a and c).

f. Scan-sweep: The probe can be moved proximally and distally on Lnx and Sax to trace the tendon from middle anterolateral aspect of the leg as it travels along the dorsum of the foot to insert on base of distal phalanx of great toe.

g. Dynamic testing: The great toe is brought into dorsiflexion and plantarflexion to assess the integrity of the tendon.

3. *Extensor Digitorum Longus (EDL) tendon and muscle.*

a. Patient Position: lying supine on table with foot free at distal edge of the table.

b. Examiner Position: seated in front of the patient.

c. Probe Placement: Sax lateral to midline at the level of the ankle joint.

d. Bony Acoustic Landmark(s): distal tibia, distal fibula, talus.

e. Target: The EDL tendon can be identified as the most lateral tendon at the anterior ankle joint region and appears as a fibrillary structure on Lnx and as a hyperechoic structure with speckled pattern appearance on Sax (Fig. 7.1a and d).

f. Scan-sweep: The probe can be moved proximally and distally on Lnx and Sax to trace the tendon from anterolateral aspect of the leg as it travels along the dorsum of the foot to divide just distal to the talus neck into four slips that continue traveling on the dorsal aspect to insert onto the middle and distal phalanges of the second through fifth toes.

g. Dynamic testing: The toes are brought into dorsiflexion and plantarflexion to assess the integrity of the tendon.

4. *Peroneus Tertius.*

a. Patient Position: lying supine on table with foot free at distal edge of the table.

b. Examiner Position: seated in front of the patient.

c. Probe Placement: Sax lateral to midline at the level of the ankle joint.

d. Bony Acoustic Landmark(s): distal tibia, distal fibula, talus.

e. Target: The peroneus tertius muscle might be absent. If present, it will be found just lateral to the EDL, running adjacent to it or in the same synovial sheath.

f. Scan-sweep: The probe can be moved proximally and distally on Sax and Lnx to trace the tendon as it inserts on the lateral cuboid or base of fifth metatarsal.

g. Dynamic testing: The foot is brought into inversion and eversion to assess the integrity of the tendon.

5. *Superior and Inferior Extensor Retinaculum.*

a. Patient Position: lying supine on table with foot free at distal edge of the table.

b. Examiner Position: seated in front of the patient.

c. Probe Placement: Sax midline at the level of the ankle joint.

d. Bony Acoustic Landmark(s): distal tibia, distal fibula, talus.

e. Target: The retinacula can be identified as fibrous bands with echogenic appearance stretching horizontally superficial to the extensor tendons.

f. Scan-sweep: The probe can be moved medially and laterally on Sax to trace the retinacula from anteromedial aspect of the ankle as they travel to their insertion points. The superior retinaculum spans from medial aspect of the tibia to the distal fibula (Fig. 7.1a). The inferior retinaculum is a Y-shaped ligament that inserts at the calcaneus, medial malleolus, and talus.

g. Dynamic testing: The foot is brought into dorsiflexion and plantarflexion to assess the integrity of the ligaments.

6. *Deep Peroneal Nerve and Dorsalis Pedis Artery.*

a. Patient Position: lying supine on table with foot free at distal edge of the table.

b. Examiner Position: seated in front of the patient.

c. Probe Placement: Sax lateral to midline at the level of the ankle joint.

d. Bony Acoustic Landmark(s): distal tibia, distal fibula, talus.

e. Target: The deep peroneal nerve and dorsalis pedis artery can be identified deeper to and between the EDL and EHL tendons at the level of the ankle joint (Fig. 7.2).

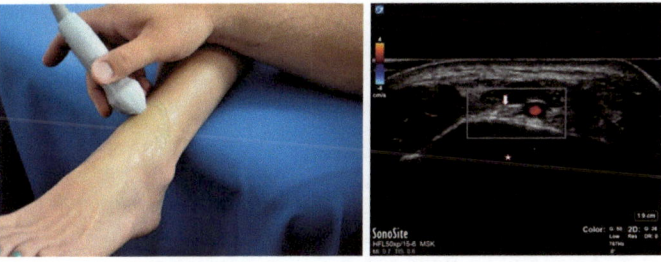

Fig. 7.2 Deep Peroneal Nerve and Dorsalis Pedis Artery. Sax view of transducer placement and corresponding ultrasound images. Deep peroneal nerve (down arrow), dorsalis pedis artery (red), and distal tibia (star)

    f. Scan-sweep: The probe can be moved proximally and distally on Lnx and Sax to trace the nerve and artery. Doppler function can be applied to differentiate the artery from the nearby vein. Light compression with the probe can also be applied to collapse the vein.

7. *Anterior Inferior Tibiofibular Ligament (AITFL).*

    a. Patient Position: lying supine on table with foot free at distal edge of the table, foot placed in inversion.

    b. Examiner Position: seated in front of the patient.

    c. Probe Placement: placed at distal end of lateral malleolus at a 45 degrees angle with the shaft of the fibula, at the level of the ankle joint, aiming proximally at the distal tibia.

    d. Bony Acoustic Landmark(s): distal tibia, distal fibula, talus.

    e. Target: The AITFL can be identified as a moderately thick echoic band at the anterior aspect of the joint (Fig. 7.3).

    f. Dynamic testing: The ankle joint is brought into eversion and dorsiflexion or external rotation to stress the ligament and assess its integrity.

8. *Anterior Joint Recess and Capsule.*

    a. Patient Position: lying supine on table with foot free at distal edge of the table.

    b. Examiner Position: seated in front of the patient.

    c. Probe Placement: Lnx midline at the level of the ankle joint.

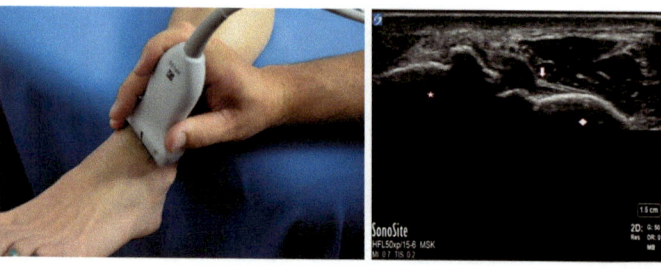

Fig. 7.3 Anterior Inferior Tibiofibular Ligament (AITFL). Lnx view of transducer placement and corresponding ultrasound images. Tibia (star), fibula (diamond) and AITFL (down arrow) can be seen

d. Bony Acoustic Landmark(s): distal tibia, distal fibula, talus.
e. Target: The anterior joint recess can be identified deeper to the extensor tendons and neurovascular structures.
f. Scan-sweep: The probe can be moved medially and laterally over the joint for complete assessment.
g. Dynamic testing: The joint can be brought through dorsiflexion and plantarflexion, eversion and inversion, and the recess can be assessed for additional fluid collection during these maneuvers.

Notes
1. Tendons are traced proximally and distally as clinically indicated.
2. Dynamic assessment of the anterior inferior tibiofibular ligament may be performed by an external rotation stress test, a squeeze test, or weight bearing.

Medial Ankle Region

9. *Posterior Tibialis Tendon and Muscle.*
    a. Patient Position: lying supine on table with leg externally rotated and foot free at distal edge of the table.
    b. Examiner Position: seated next to the patient.

    c. Probe Placement: Sax behind the medial malleolus at 45 degrees with the shaft of the tibia, at the level of the ankle joint.

    d. Bony Acoustic Landmark(s): medial malleolus.

    e. Target: The posterior tibialis is the largest and most anterior tendon in the medial region of the ankle, and can be seen as a fibrillary structure on Lnx and as a hyperechoic structure with speckled pattern appearance on Sax (Fig. 7.4a and b).

    f. Scan-sweep: The probe can be moved proximally and distally to trace the tendon as it runs below the medial malleolus before fanning out into multiple slips and inserting on the navicular and the rest of the tarsal bones (except talus, and second through fourth metatarsals). Doppler function can be utilized to assess the tendon for inflammatory conditions.

    g. Dynamic testing: The foot can be brought through inversion and eversion to assess for the integrity of the tendon.

10. *Flexor Digitorum Longus (FDL) Tendon and Muscle.*

    a. Patient Position: lying supine on table with leg externally rotated and foot free at distal edge of the table.

    b. Examiner Position: seated next to the patient.

    c. Probe Placement: Sax behind the medial malleolus at 45 degrees with the shaft of the tibia, at the level of the ankle joint.

    d. Bony Acoustic Landmark(s): medial malleolus.

    e. Target: The FDL is situated just posterior to and thinner than the posterior tibialis tendon, and can be seen as a fibrillary structure on Lnx and as a hyperechoic structure with speckled pattern appearance on Sax (Fig. 7.4a).

    f. Scan-sweep: The probe can be moved proximally and distally to trace the tendon as it runs below the medial malleolus along the inner aspect of the sustentaculum tali and inserts plantarly at the second through fifth distal phalanges.

    g. Dynamic testing: The patient is asked to flex and extend the toes to assess for the integrity and motion of the tendon.

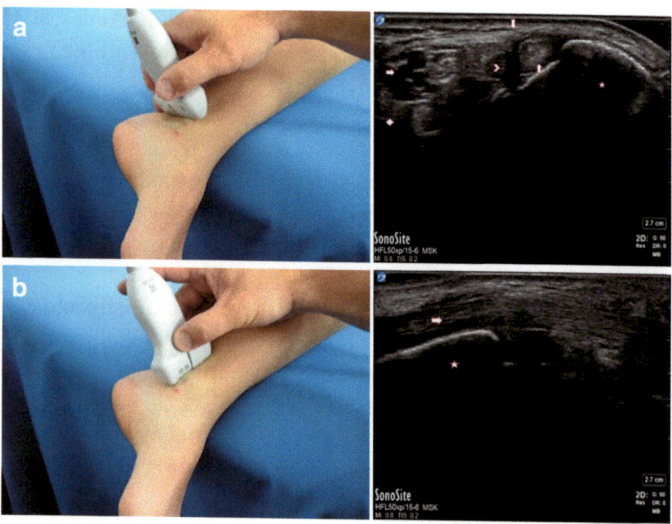

Fig. 7.4 Tibialis Posterior (TP), Flexor Digitorum Longus (FDL), Flexor Hallucis Longus (FHL) Tendons and Muscles. TP, FHL, and FDL tendons (Sax and Lnx). Sax view (**a**) for all 3 tendons at the posteromedial ankle and Lnx view for TP (**b**) of transducer placement and corresponding ultrasound images. (**a**) TP (up arrow), FDL (chevron), FHL (diamond), neurovacscular bundle (horizontal arrow), tibia (star), and flexor retinaculum (down arrows) can be seen. (**b**) Tibia (star) and TP (horizontal arrow)

11. *Posterior Tibial Nerve, Tibial Artery and Veins, and Medial and Lateral Plantar Nerves.*
    a. Patient Position: lying supine on table with leg externally rotated and foot free at distal edge of the table.
    b. Examiner Position: seated next to the patient.
    c. Probe Placement: Sax behind the medial malleolus at 45 degrees with the shaft of the tibia, at the level of the ankle joint.
    d. Bony Acoustic Landmark(s): medial malleolus.
    e. Target: The neurovascular bundle (posterior tibial nerve, tibial artery, and tibial veins) can be identified adjacent to FDL and superficial to the FHL tendons. The posterior tibial nerve has a honeycomb appearance on Sax, while the veins are collapsible with pressure applied through the probe (Fig. 7.5).

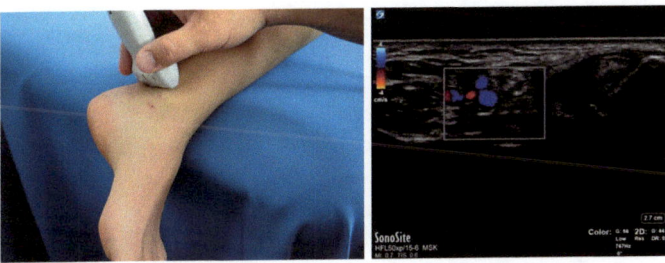

Fig. 7.5 Posterior Tibial Nerve, Tibial Artery and Veins. Sax view of transducer placement and corresponding ultrasound image

f. Scan-sweep: The probe can be moved proximally and distally to trace the nerve as it divides into its medial and lateral plantar nerves branches. Doppler function can be applied to differentiate the veins from the artery.

12. *Flexor Hallucis Longus (FHL) Tendon and Muscle.*

a. Patient Position: lying supine on table with leg externally rotated and foot free at distal edge of the table.

b. Examiner Position: seated next to the patient.

c. Probe Placement: Sax behind the medial malleolus at 45 degrees with the shaft of the tibia, at the level of the ankle joint.

d. Bony Acoustic Landmark(s): medial malleolus.

e. Target: The FHL is situated deep and posterior to the rest of the tendons in the medial ankle region just posterior to and thinner than the posterior tibialis tendon, and can be seen as a fibrillary structure on Lnx and as a hyperechoic structure with speckled pattern appearance on Sax (Fig. 7.4a).

f. Scan-sweep: The probe can be moved proximally and distally to trace the tendon as it runs in the plantar plane under the sustentaculum tali and intersecting the FDL tendon to continue to its insertion point at the great toe distal phalanx.

g. Dynamic testing: The patient is asked to flex and extend the great toe to assess for the integrity and motion of the tendon.

13. *Deltoid Ligament and Medial Tibiotalar Joint.*
    a. Patient Position: lying supine on table with leg externally rotated and foot free at distal edge of the table.
    b. Examiner Position: seated next to the patient.
    c. Probe Placement: Sax on the medial malleolus at the level of the ankle joint.
    d. Bony Acoustic Landmark(s): medial malleolus, talus, calcaneus, navicular.
    e. Target: The probe is anchored on the medial malleolus as the various portions of the deltoid ligament are identified. The deeper short band inserts on the medial talus. The superficial portion is delta shaped and attaches to the navicular, talus, and the calcaneus (Fig. 7.6a and b).
    f. Dynamic testing: Dorsiflexion of the foot will allow better examination of the posterior aspect of the ligament, while the tibionavicular portion will best be seen with the foot positioned in neutral.
14. *Flexor Retinaculum.*
    a. Patient Position: lying supine on table with leg externally rotated and foot free at distal edge of the table.
    b. Examiner Position: seated next to the patient.
    c. Probe Placement: on the medial malleolus at the level of the ankle joint with the distal portion pointing posteriorly towards the medial calcaneal region.
    d. Bony Acoustic Landmark(s): medial malleolus, calcaneus.
    e. Target: The flexor retinaculum will appear as a thin echogenic band overlying the tendons of the medial ankle region and spanning from the medial malleolus to the calcaneus.

Notes
1. Tendons are traced proximally and distally as clinically indicated.
2. To reduce anisotropy, the ankle is placed in plantarflexion to reduce the curvature of the tendons and nerves in the perimalleolar region.

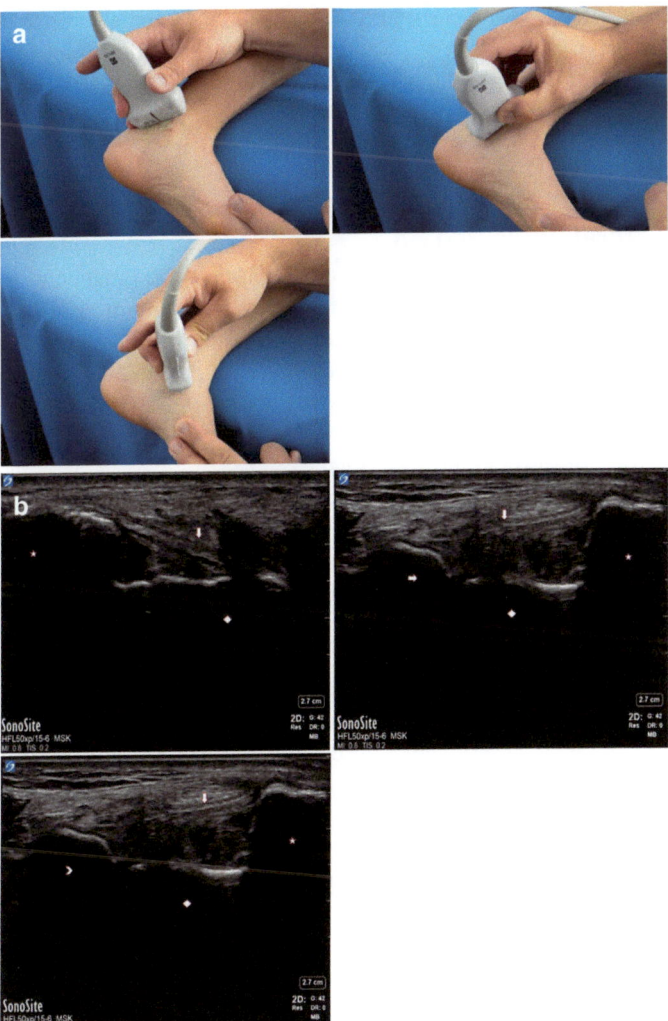

Fig. 7.6 Deltoid Ligament and Medial Tibiotalar Joint. Deltoid ligament and underlying medial tibiotalar joint views (**a**) for transducer placement and (**b**) corresponding ultrasound images. (**b**) Tibia (star), Talus (diamond), Navicular (horizontal arrow), Calcaneus (chevron), and Deltoid ligament (down arrows) can be seen

3. Although not consistently visualized, the medial calcaneal nerve typically arises from the tibial nerve and courses into the subcutaneous tissue of the medial heel.
4. Distal examination of the posterior tibialis may include assessment of os naviculare and the spring ligament.

Lateral Ankle Region

15. *Peroneus Longus and Brevis Tendons and Muscles.*
    a. Patient Position: lying supine on table with leg internally rotated and foot free at distal edge of the table.
    b. Examiner Position: seated next to the patient.
    c. Probe Placement: on Sax behind the lateral malleolus at the level of the ankle joint.
    d. Bony Acoustic Landmark(s): Lateral malleolus, calcaneus.
    e. Target: The peroneal brevis tendon can be identified as the thinner tendon closer to the posterior aspect of the lateral malleolus, while the peroneal longus is a larger tendon located posterior to it. The tendons will be seen as fibrillary structures on Lnx and as hyperechoic structures with speckled pattern appearance on Sax (Fig. 7.7a and b).
    f. Scan-sweep: The probe can be moved proximally and distally on Sax and Lnx to trace the tendons proximally, where the myotendinous junction of the peroneus brevis can be identified more distally compared to that of the peroneus longus. As the tendons run below the lateral malleolus, at the level of the lateral aspect of the calcaneus, the peroneus brevis is identified superior to the peroneus longus tendon before reaching its insertion at the base of fifth metatarsal. The peroneus longus can be traced to its insertion as it travels on the inferolateral aspect of the cuboid to its insertion on the base of the first and second metatarsals.
    g. Dynamic testing: The foot can be brought through inversion and eversion to assess for the integrity of the tendons. At the level of the ankle, the tendons are assessed for subluxation from the posterior aspect of the lateral malleolus.

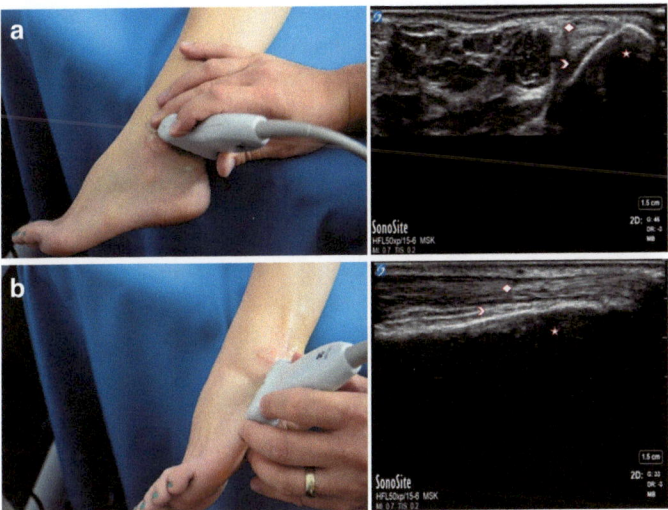

Fig. 7.7 Peroneus Longus and Brevis Tendons and Muscles. Peroneus Longus and Brevis (Sax and Lnx). Sax view (**a**) and Lnx view (**b**) of transducer placement and corresponding ultrasound images. Peroneus Longus (diamond) and Brevis (chevron) and distal fibula (star) are highlighted

16. *Superior and Inferior Peroneal Retinaculum.*
    a. Patient Position: lying supine on table with leg internally rotated and foot free at distal edge of the table.
    b. Examiner Position: seated next to the patient.
    c. Probe Placement: on Sax behind the lateral malleolus at the level of the ankle joint.
    d. Bony Acoustic Landmark(s): lateral malleolus, calcaneus.
    e. Target: The superior peroneal retinaculum is identified as it extends from the lateral malleolus to outer surface of calcaneus, while the lower retinaculum can be seen as it travels from the lateral aspect of the inferior extensor retinaculum to the calcaneus, distal to the ankle joint level.
    f. Dynamic testing: The patient is asked to dorsiflex and evert the foot to assess for the integrity of the retinacula.

17. *Anterior Talofibular Ligament (ATFL).*
    a. Patient Position: lying supine on table with leg internally rotated and foot inverted, plantarflexed, and free at distal edge of the table.
    b. Examiner Position: seated next to the patient.
    c. Probe Placement: on Lnx at the lateral malleolus at the level of the ankle joint, perpendicular to the shaft axis of the tibia.
    d. Bony Acoustic Landmark(s): lateral malleolus, talus.
    e. Target: The ATFL can be identified as it extends from the anterior portion of the lateral malleolus to the talar neck (Fig. 7.8).
    f. Dynamic testing: With the foot in plantarflexion, an anteriorly directed force is placed on the posterior aspect of the foot and the fibula-talus distance is assessed for any gaps to assess for the integrity of the ligament.

18. *Calcaneofibular Ligament (CFL), Lateral Tibiotalar joint, and Posterior Subtalar joint.*
    a. Patient Position: lying supine on table with leg internally rotated and foot inverted, dorsiflexed, and free at distal edge of the table.
    b. Examiner Position: seated next to the patient.
    c. Probe Placement: on Lnx with proximal aspect of the probe at the lateral malleolus at the level of the ankle joint, parallel to the shaft axis of the tibia.

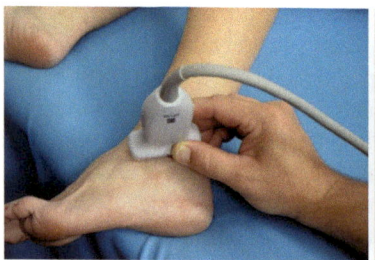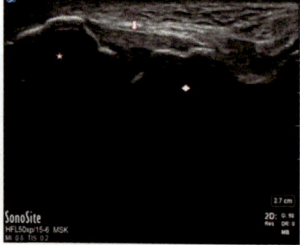

Fig. 7.8 Anterior Talofibular Ligament (ATFL). ATFL Lnx view of transducer placement and corresponding ultrasound image. Talus (diamond), Fibula (star), and ATFL (arrow) are highlighted

d. Bony Acoustic Landmark(s): lateral malleolus, calcaneus.

e. Target: The CFL can be identified deep to the peroneal tendons, as it extends from the tip of the lateral malleolus to the lateral aspect of the calcaneus. The lateral aspect of the tibiotalar joint is identified deeper to the CFL as it crosses the fibulotalar space, while the posterior subtalar joint can be identified deeper to the ligament as it approaches its insertion on the calcaneus (Fig. 7.9).

f. Dynamic testing: With the foot in dorsiflexion, an anteriorly directed force is placed on the posterior aspect of the foot and the fibula-calcaneus distance is assessed for any gaps to assess for the integrity of the ligament.

19. *Posterior Talofibular Ligament (PTFL).*

a. Patient Position: lying supine on table with leg internally rotated and foot inverted and free at distal edge of the table.

b. Examiner Position: seated next to the patient.

c. Probe Placement: on Lnx with proximal aspect of the probe at the lateral malleolus at the level of the ankle joint, parallel to the shaft axis of the tibia.

d. Bony Acoustic Landmark(s): lateral malleolus, talus.

e. Target: The PTFL can be identified distal to the PITFL as it extends from the posterior aspect of lateral malleolus to the posterior aspect of the talus (Fig. 7.10).

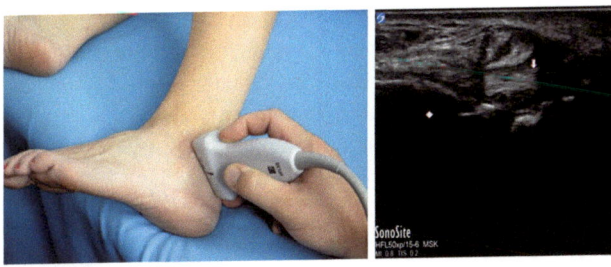

Fig. 7.9 Calcanofibular Ligament (CFL). CFL Lnx view of transducer placement and corresponding ultrasound image. Calcaneus (diamond), Fibula (star), and CFL (arrow) are highlighted

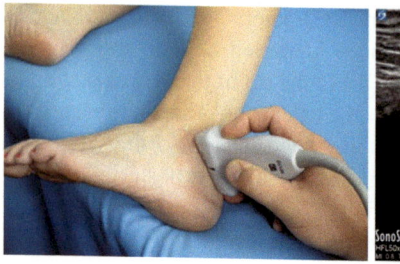 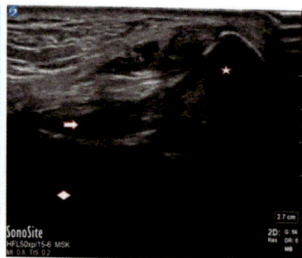

Fig. 7.10 Posterior Talofibular Ligament (PTFL). PTFL Lnx view of transducer placement and corresponding ultrasound image. Calcaneus (diamond), Fibula (star), and PTFL (arrow) are highlighted

Notes

1. Tendons are traced proximally and distally as clinically indicated.
2. To reduce anisotropy, the ankle is placed in plantarflexion to reduce the curvature of the tendons and nerves in the perimalleolar region.
3. The sural nerve is identified in the interval between the fibularis (peroneal) tendons anteriorly and the Achilles tendon posteriorly, lying directly adjacent to the small saphenous vein.
4. Distal examination of the fibularis (peroneus) longus assessment for an os peroneum embedded in the longus tendon at the level of the lateral cuboid.
5. Fibularis/peroneal tendon subluxation may be elicited by active or resisted dorsiflexion-eversion, or circumduction.
6. The lateral recess of the posterior subtalar joint is visualized deep to the calcaneofibular ligament.
7. Dynamic assessment for anterior ankle instability may be performed using the anterior drawer test.

Posterior Ankle Region

20. *Achilles Tendon, Paratenon, and Plantaris Tendon.*
    a. Patient Position: lying prone on table with foot free at distal edge of the table.

b. Examiner Position: seated next to the patient.

c. Probe Placement: on Lnx midline at the posterior aspect of the leg, in line with the axis of the tibia.

d. Bony Acoustic Landmark(s): posterior malleolus, calcaneus.

e. Target: The Achilles tendon can be identified as the most superficial tendon on Lnx. On Sax examination, the tendon has a crescentic appearance with a concave anterior aspect. The plantaris tendon can be identified as it runs just medial to the Achilles tendon. The tendons will be seen as fibrillary structures on Lnx and as hyperechoic structures with speckled pattern appearance on Sax. The paratenon can be identified medially and laterally to the Achilles tendon (Fig. 7.11a and b).

f. Scan-sweep: The Achilles tendon is followed on Sax and Lnx from its myotendinous junction to its insertion on the calcaneus. On Sax, the probe is moved laterally and medially at different level to assess the tendon along its width. The plantaris tendon is traced on Lnx and Sax proximally to the muscle origin from supracondylar ridge of the femur, and to its insertion distally on the calcaneus or the Achilles tendon. Doppler function can be used to assess for hypervascularity indicating and inflammatory process.

g. Dynamic testing: The foot can be brought through active dorsiflexion and plantarflexion, or the calf muscles can be squeezed by the examiner to assess the integrity of the tendon.

21. *Retrocalcaneal and Retro-Achilles Bursa.*

a. Patient Position: lying prone on table with foot free at distal edge of the table.

b. Examiner Position: seated next to the patient.

c. Probe Placement: on Sax midline at the posterior aspect of the leg, in line with the axis of the tibia, minimal pressure applied.

d. Bony Acoustic Landmark(s): posterior malleolus, calcaneus.

e. Target: The retro-Achilles bursa is subcutaneous and is located over the distal aspect of the Achilles tendon. The

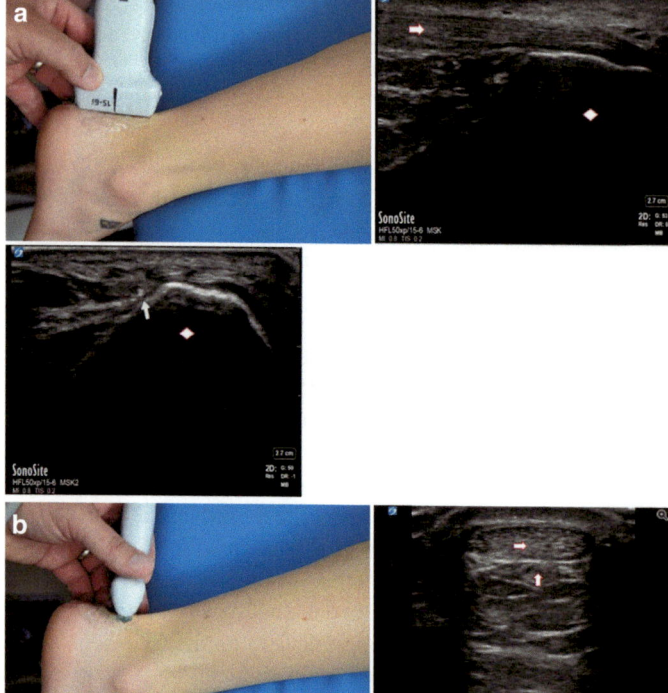

Fig. 7.11 Achilles and Plantaris Tendons. Achilles and Plantaris tendons (Sax and Lnx). Lnx view (**a**) and Sax views (**b**) of transducer placement and corresponding ultrasound images. Achilles (horizontal arrow), Calcaneus (chevron), and Plantaris (up arrow) can be seen

retrocalcaneal bursa can be identified on the brow of the calcaneus deep to attachment of the Achilles tendon.

22. *Posterior Tibiotalar and Subtalar Joints.*
    a. Patient Position: lying prone on table with foot free at distal edge of the table.
    b. Examiner Position: seated next to the patient.

c. Probe Placement: on Lnx midline at the posterior aspect of the leg, in line with the axis of the tibia.

d. Bony Acoustic Landmark(s): posterior malleolus, calcaneus.

e. Target: The FHL tendon can be identified running deep to the Achilles tendon. Deeper to the FHL the posterior tibiotalar and the more distal subtalar joints can be identified, and assessed for effusion (Fig. 7.12a).

f. Dynamic testing: The ankle can be brought through dorsiflexion and plantarflexion, and inversion and eversion to assess for joints effusion (Fig. 7.12b and c).

23. *Plantar Fascia.*

a. Patient Position: lying prone on table with foot free at distal edge of the table.

b. Examiner Position: seated facing the patient's foot.

c. Probe Placement: on Lnx at just medial to midline at posterior aspect of the heel.

d. Bony Acoustic Landmark(s): calcaneus.

e. Target: The plantar fascia can be identified as it originates from the medial aspect of the calcaneus (Fig. 7.13a and b).

f. Scan-sweep: The plantar fascia is followed distally while sweeping medially and laterally. Doppler function can be used to assess for hypervascularity.

Notes

1. Examination for superficial bursa may require a standoff pad or heaping gel on the skin to minimize transducer pressure and the possibility of a false negative examination.

2. Dynamic assessment of the Achilles tendon is performed using passive ankle plantarflexion and dorsiflexion. In the setting of Achilles tendon rupture, tendon apposition during plantarflexion suggests the option of non-operative treatment in appropriate clinical circumstances.

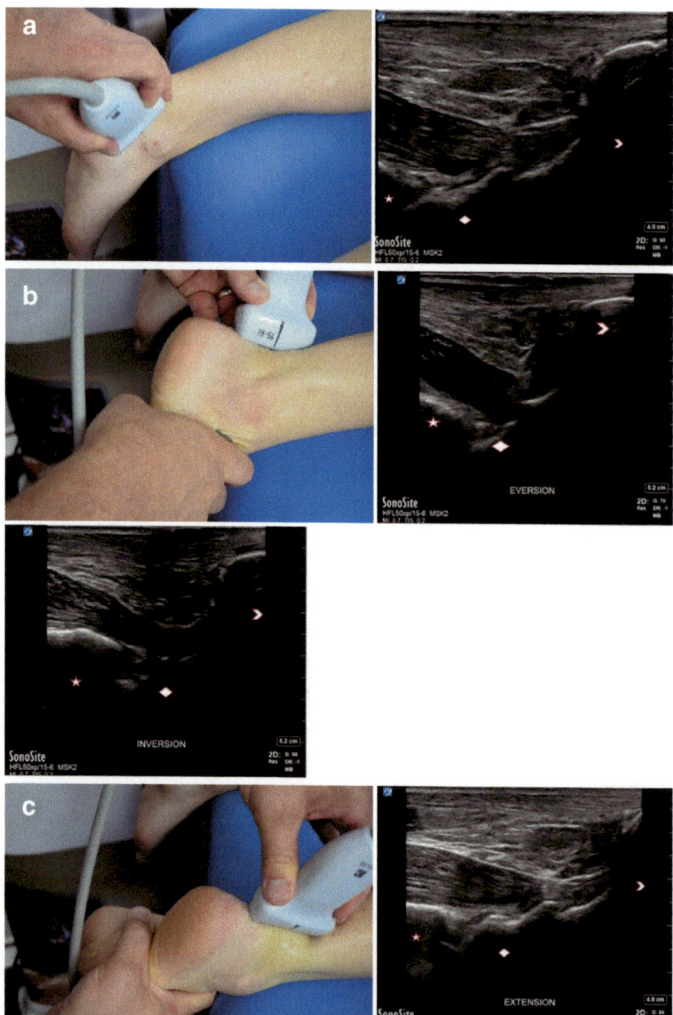

Fig. 7.12 Posterior Tibiotalar and Subtalar Joints. Posterior tibiotalar and subtalar joint spaces views of transducer placement and corresponding ultrasound images. Tibia (star), Talus (diamond) and Calcaneus (chevron can be seen with the foot in neutral (**a**), inversion and eversion (**b**), and plantarflexion (**c**)

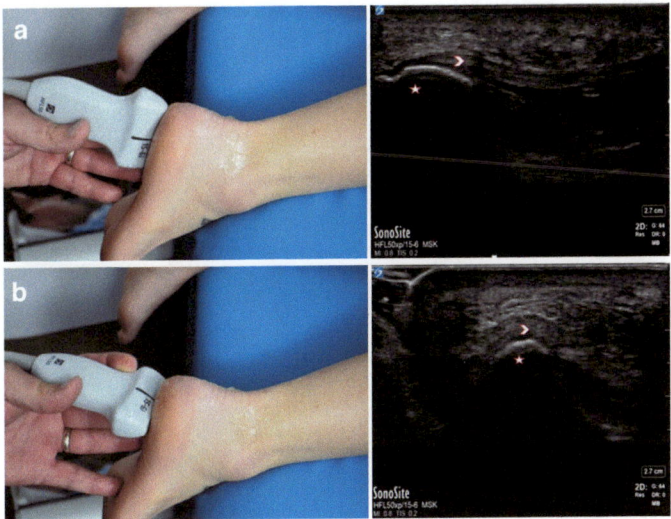

Fig. 7.13 Plantar Fascia. Plantar fascia Lnx (**a**) and Sax (**b**) views of transducer placement and corresponding ultrasound images. Calcaneus (star), and Fascia (chevron) can be seen

Foot Region

24. *Intermetatarsal Space, Morton's Neuroma, and Ultrasonographic Mulder's click (as indicated).*
    a. Patient Position: lying supine on table with foot free at distal edge of the table in neutral flexion.
    b. Examiner Position: seated next to the patient.
    c. Probe Placement: high frequency on Lnx at the dorsum of the foot.
    d. Bony Acoustic Landmark(s): metatarsals, tarsal bones.
    e. Target: The intermetatarsal spaces are assessed in Sax and Lnx (Fig. 7.14a).
    f. Dynamic testing: As the intermetatarsal space is assessed, the examiner applies dorsally directed pressure over the plantar aspect of the foot, widening the intermetatarsal space and facilitating examination of the various structures (Fig. 7.14b). This maneuver assists in the differentia-

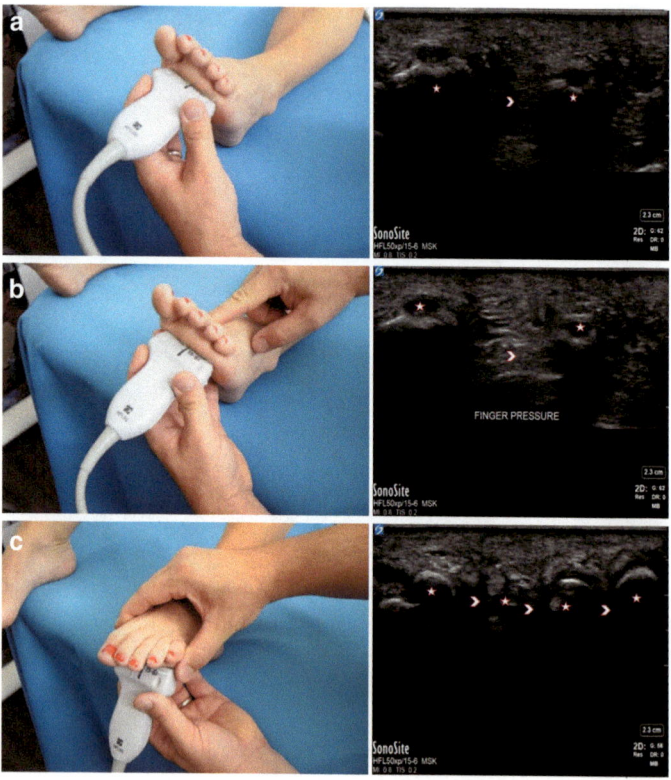

Fig. 7.14 Intermetatarsal Space, Morton's Neuroma, and Ultrasonographic Mulder's click (as indicated). Intermetatarsal space Sax views of transducer placement and corresponding ultrasound images. Metatarsals (star), and Intermetatarsal space containing nerve (chevron) can be seen with the foot in neutral (**a**). The Web-space tenderness test (**b**) and the Mulder sonographic test (**c**) are highlighted

tion of Morton neuroma and intermetatarsal bursitis. The Mulder sonographic test can be performed in equivocal cases by scanning the plantar aspect of the forefoot as lateral compression forces are applied to the metatarsal heads and will reveal a plantarly displacing Morton neuroma and a click if the condition is present (Fig. 7.14c).

Notes

1. A dorsal approach is often favored due to the presence of plantar callous.

25. *Metatarsophalangeal Joints (MTPJ).*
    a. Patient Position: lying supine on table with foot free at distal edge of the table in neutral flexion.
    b. Examiner Position: seated next to the patient.
    c. Probe Placement: high frequency on Lnx at the level of the metatarsal of interest.
    d. Bony Acoustic Landmark(s): metatarsals, proximal phalanges.
    e. Target: MTPJ of various toes can be assessed for effusion. The extensor tendons can be identified as thin hyperechoic fibrillar bands running into the subcutaneous tissue superficial to the joints (Fig. 7.15a and b).
    f. Dynamic testing: As the intermetatarsal space is assessed, the examiner applies dorsally directed pressure over the plantar aspect of the foot. The toes can be brought through flexion and extension to assess for any abnormalities.

26. *Interphalangeal Joints (ITPJ).*
    a. Patient Position: lying supine on table with foot free at distal edge of the table in neutral flexion.
    b. Examiner Position: seated next to the patient.
    c. Probe Placement: high frequency on Lnx at the level of the toe of interest.
    d. Bony Acoustic Landmark(s): phalanges.
    e. Target: ITPJ of various toes can be assessed for effusion. The extensor tendons can be identified as thin hyperechoic fibrillar bands running into the subcutaneous tissue superficial to the joints (Fig. 7.16).
    f. Dynamic testing: The toes can be brought through flexion and extension to assess for any abnormalities.

Notes

1. Examination Extended to Other Joints As Clinically Indicated

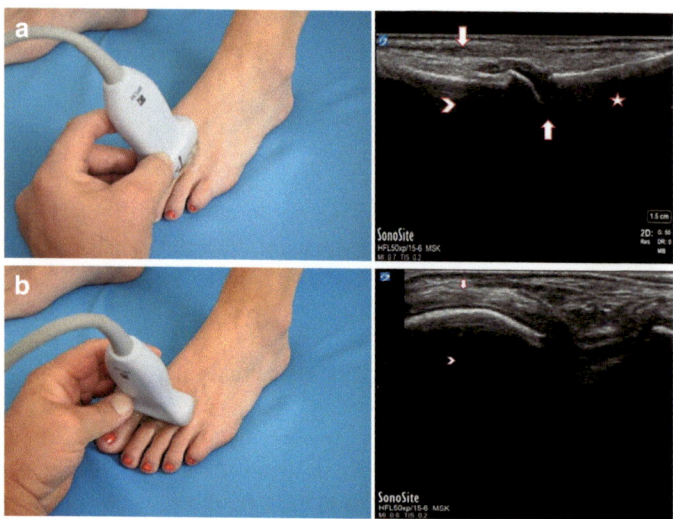

Fig. 7.15 Metatarsophalangeal Joints (MTPJ). MTPJ Lnx (**a**) and Sax (**b**) views of transducer placement and corresponding ultrasound images. Metatarsal (chevron), proximal phalanx (star), MTP joint space and joint capsule (up arrow) and extensor digitorum (down arrow)

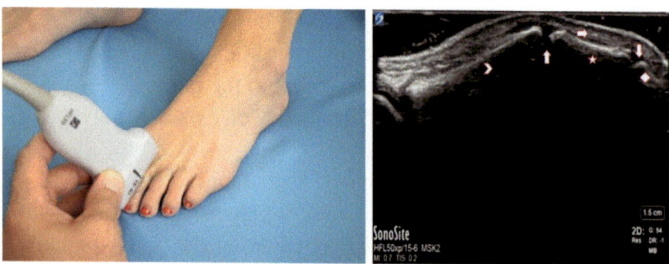

Fig. 7.16 Interphalangeal Joints (ITPJ). ITPJ Lnx views of transducer placement and corresponding ultrasound image. Proximal phalanx (chevron), middle phalanx (star), extensor digitorum (horizontal arrow), and distal phalanx (diamond) proximal and distal interphalangeal joint spaces (up and down arrow, respectively) and joint capsule (up arrow)

Resources

AIUM Practice Guidelines for the Performance of the Musculo-skeletal Ultrasound Examination, 2012.

American Institute of Ultrasound In Medicine (www.aium.org)

European Society of Skeletal Radiology (www.essr.org)

Jacobson JA. Fundamentals of Musculoskeletal Ultrasound, 2nd ed., Saunders Elsevier; Philadelphia; 2013. ISBN 978-1-4557-3818-2.

Bianchi S, Martinoli C. Ultrasound of the Musculoskeletal System. New York: Springer, 2007, ISBN 978-3-540-42267-9, 974 pp.

O'Neill J (ed.). Musculoskeletal Ultrasound: Anatomy and Technique. New York: Springer, 2008, ISBN 978-0-387-76609-6, 348 pp.

Kremkau F. Diagnostic Ultrasound: Principles and Instruments. 6th ed. Philadelphia, PA: WB Saunders; 2002:428.

© The Editor(s) (if applicable) and The Author(s), under exclusive license to Springer Nature Switzerland AG 2022
M. M. El-Othmani et al., *Sports Medicine and Musculoskeletal Ultrasound*, https://doi.org/10.1007/978-3-031-11764-0

Index

© The Editor(s) (if applicable) and The Author(s), under exclusive license to Springer Nature Switzerland AG 2022
M. M. El-Othmani et al., *Sports Medicine and Musculoskeletal Ultrasound*, https://doi.org/10.1007/978-3-031-11764-0